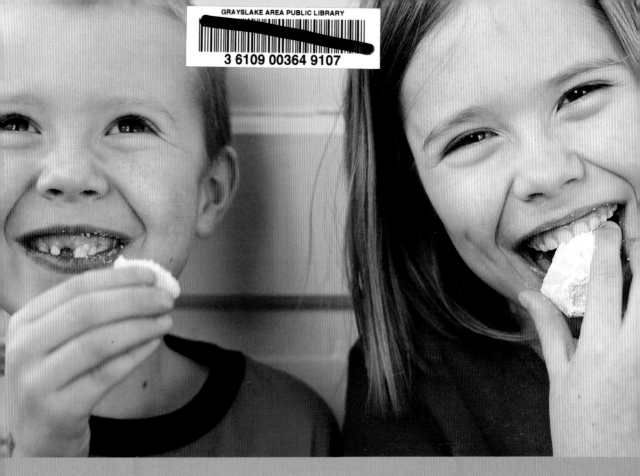

GRAYSLAKE AREA PUBLIC LIBRARY

3 6109 00364 9107

NO LONGER OWNED BY
GRAYSLAKE PUBLIC LIBRARY

THE
Food Allergy Mama's
BAKING BOOK

P9-BZD-187

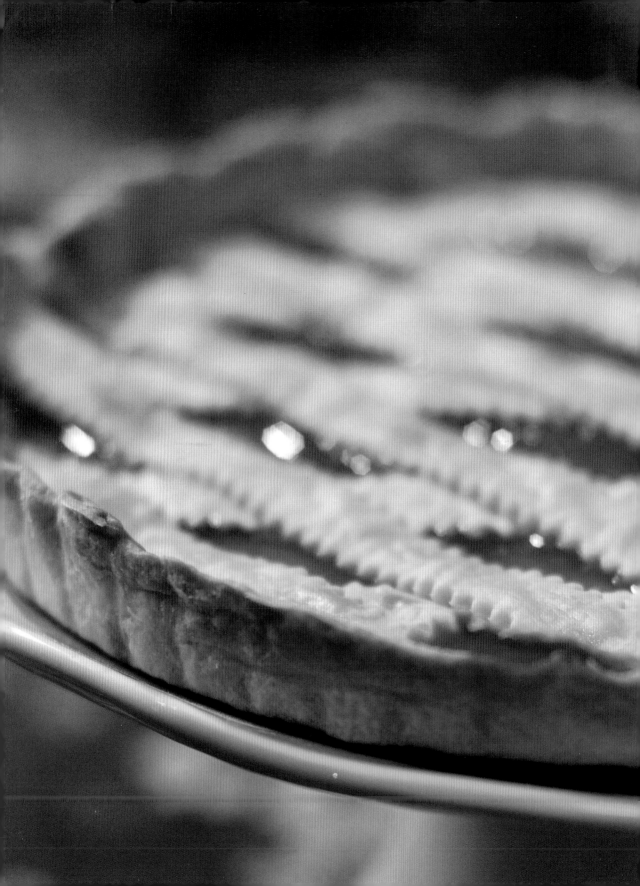

THE
Food Allergy Mama's
BAKING BOOK

Great Dairy, Egg, and Nut-Free Treats for the Whole Family

KELLY RUDNICKI

Surrey Books
Chicago

GRAYSLAKE AREA PUBLIC LIBRARY
100 Library Lane
Grayslake, IL 60030

641.5631
RUD
To

Copyright © 2009 Kelly Rudnicki

All rights reserved. No part of this book may be repro-
duced or transmitted in any form or by any means, elec-
tronic or mechanical, including photocopying, recording,
or by any information storage and retrieval system, without express written permission from the publisher.

Printed in Malaysia.

All photographs by Robert Knapp.
Design by Brandtner Design.

Library of Congress Cataloging-in-Publication Data

Rudnicki, Kelly.
 The food allergy mama's baking book : great dairy, egg,
and nut-free treats for the whole family / Kelly Rudnicki.
     p. cm.
 Summary: "Nut-, dairy-, and egg-free recipes for home
baking. Includes tricks and tips for families dealing with
food allergies"--Provided by publisher.
 Includes index.
 ISBN-13: 978-1-57284-102-4 (pbk.)
 ISBN-10: 1-57284-102-8 (pbk.)
 1. Food allergy in children.--Diet therapy--Recipes. 2.
Baking. I. Title.
 RJ386.5.R83 2009
 641.5'63--dc22
                        2009011930

10 12 13
10 9 8 7 6 5 4 3 2

Surrey Books is an imprint of Agate Publishing. Agate
books are available in bulk at discount prices. For more
information, go to agatepublishing.com

3 6109 00364 9107

Table of Contents

To my mother, who inspired my love for baking in the first place.

Forewords

As a mother of two children with life-threatening food allergies, I have spent the last fifteen years trying to protect my sons *and* provide variety and nutritional balance in their diets. Those of you who have picked up this book can surely relate to the challenges we face as parents and providers for food-allergic families. More than ten years ago, my friend, Anne Thompson, and I started a support group for others like ourselves—Mothers of Children Having Allergies (MOCHA). We felt the need to connect with other families in the Chicago area to share what we were all learning as new initiates to the foreign world of food allergies.

It was at one of our MOCHA meetings that I met Kelly Rudnicki and recognized her enthusiasm and commitment to advancing the cause of food allergy research while providing practical day-to-day assistance to those in the trenches. Not only has she worked for many years to protect and provide for her own food-allergic son, but she has also had the inspiration and dedication to share with the rest of us many of her time-tested recipes and suggestions.

Is it possible to have too many options when feeding our families their very limited diets? I don't think so. I salivate as I read this cookbook full of goodies like Apple House Cinnamon Doughnuts, Chocolate Chip Bars, and Lemon Granitas. I especially appreciate that Kelly included specific brands of ingredients and very detailed lists of substitutions. The reader will find this information both helpful and inspiring.

While those of us with food-allergic children often try to focus our celebrations around themes other than food, the reality is that food is a vital part of fellowship, memories, and traditions. It is truly a blessing to be able to flip through this cookbook to find just the right recipe to incorporate into our special occasions and to know that not only is the recipe safe but also that the result will be delicious and memorable.

As we enjoy these recipes, the possibility of life-threatening danger still exists from even the smallest misstep. It is my passion to find a cure for this disease so that my sons, Kelly's son, and others can live their lives to the fullest, free from this threat.

Putting action behind that passion, my husband, Dave, and I founded the Food Allergy Project (FAP) as a vehicle for increasing awareness and federal funding for scientific food allergy research. Recently, FAP merged with the Food Allergy Initiative (FAI), thereby creating the largest private source of funding for food allergy research in the country. This joint endeavor serves as a voice for millions of families to call on the federal government and private sources to collaborate in search of a cure.

Currently, international research is being carried out through the Bunning Food Allergy Institute at Children's Memorial Hospital in Chicago. This study is looking for genetic indicators of food allergy in an effort to prevent the development of food allergies, as well as to find a cure for the disease. If you live in the Chicagoland area, we strongly encourage your participation in this study.

Kelly has demonstrated additional commitment to this vision by her decision to donate a portion of the proceeds from *The Food Allergy Mama's Baking Book: Great Dairy, Egg and Nut-Free Treats for the Whole Family* to help fund food allergy research. If that weren't enough, Kelly is also in training to run a marathon in Chicago with the goal of raising even more funds for food allergy research!

The efforts, energy, and enthusiasm of Kelly Rudnicki, and all the others who have worked tirelessly for the benefit of the food-allergic community, have produced results so we now have easier-to-read food labels, restaurants that accommodate food allergy requests, and schools that work to provide a safer environment for their food-allergic students. There are still many goals to accomplish and milestones to reach. We have hope for the future and, with Kelly's delicious recipes, comfort food for the food-allergic to nibble along the way!

DENISE BUNNING
COFOUNDER, FOOD ALLERGY PROJECT AND MOTHERS
OF CHILDREN HAVING ALLERGIES

As parents of three young children, we say kudos to Kelly Rudnicki. Kelly's book, *The Food Allergy Mama's Baking Book: Great Dairy, Egg and Nut-Free Treats for the Whole Family*, has modified many of our favorite, most memorable treats so they're safe for our kids.

These days, countless children diagnosed with food allergies are unable to enjoy many of the foods that make us smile. As close friends of the Rudnicki family, we've seen their son John's struggle with food allergies. When John was diagnosed, we witnessed Kelly grab her apron and spatula and turn her kitchen into a dairy, egg, and nut-free zone.

Not only are we Kelly's friends, but we also share the same commitment in our own business. Back in 1995, we started Kim and Scott's Gourmet Pretzels, and today we're proud to run a nut-free bakery that provides all-natural, nut-free soft pretzels for the frozen aisles of grocery stores, supermarket chains, coffee shops, movie theaters, and airports around the country.

Our business is inspired by moms like Kelly and kids like our nine-year-old niece, Jordyn, who also lives with severe nut, dairy, and egg allergies. We want to make sure that kids like Jordyn only have to worry about which pretzel flavor to choose (our favorites are Cheddar Jalapeño and Chocolate Crumb)—and not if it's going to make them sick.

At our pretzel twisting café, we feel it's critical to offer soy milk and a menu that includes wheat-free options so all children are included, no matter what their dietary restrictions may be. We're also working feverishly on a gluten-free pretzel line. After all, every child deserves to enjoy healthy, safe, and tasty food offerings.

We're sensitive to food allergies and conscious about what we put into our manufactured products, and now Kelly is bringing those same concepts to your kitchen. Thanks to *The Food Allergy Mama's Baking Book*, you can create delicious treats you never thought your child could enjoy.

Kelly has spent countless days in her kitchen baking, tweaking, modifying, and testing these recipes. Once you sit down with this cookbook, you won't know which recipe to make first. Each recipe sounds more delicious than the one before it (Texas Sheet Cake with the Texas Glaze makes us smile, and the Blueberry Buckle loaded with fresh fruit and topped with a crunchy streusel topping is scrumptious, too).

Grab a pen and a piece of paper, because you'll make a beeline for the grocery store with her ideas for egg, milk, and tree-nut substitutions. She even offers up some great recommendations for birthday parties, and how to make sure your child and others have fun along the way. (By the way, her Classic Chocolate Birthday Cake is a must-try.)

From the breads and doughs to the cookies and cakes, the book enables you to embrace tradition, using family recipes with the necessary modifications for food allergies. Kelly even uses her mom's Bundt pan from years ago. This book has mouthwatering tradition written all over it.

Kelly has made a difference in our lives, and she will do so for you and your loved ones who live with food allergies. Busy moms of food-allergic kids will love seeing their kids' eyes light up as they put the plates on the table. As Kelly says, "Shouldn't every kid have his cake, and eat it too?"

In her book, Kelly says she hopes "that someday, food allergy mamas everywhere will get to see the day when food allergies are a thing of the past." Until that day, we praise her for helping out all of those food allergy mamas, papas, aunts, uncles, and friends who are fortunate enough to have this delicious resource.

KIM AND SCOTT HOLSTEIN
FOUNDERS, KIM & SCOTT'S GOURMET PRETZELS

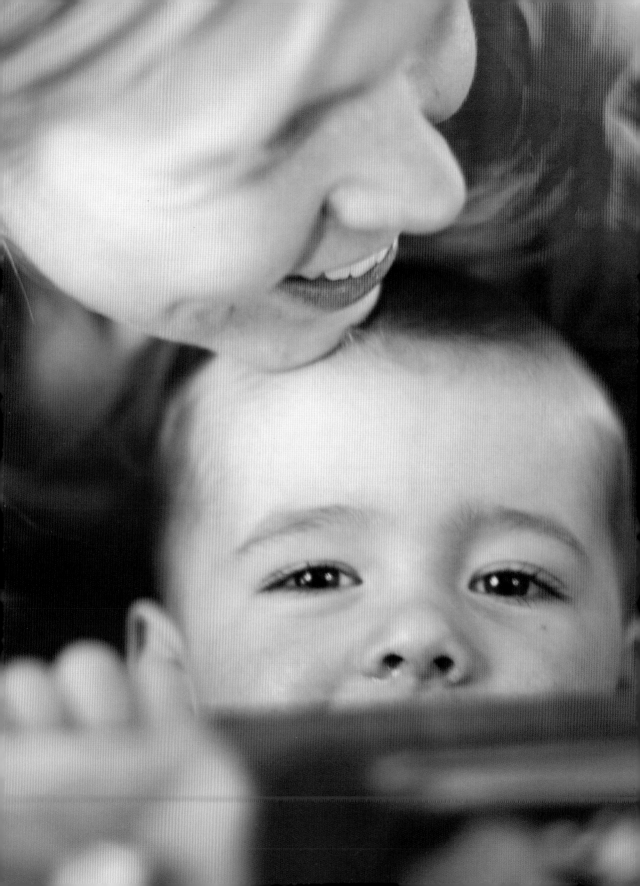

Introduction

Writing this book has been a true labor of love for me. I love to eat sweets, treats, and everything in between. When my oldest son, John, was diagnosed with life-threatening food allergies in 2003, I was dumbfounded. I had heard little about food allergies, and I didn't know any other children who suffered from them. I knew that the delicious treats I always had around the house would soon be a thing of the past, and I despaired that John would be denied the pleasures of homemade cookies, cakes, and pies.

I'll never forget the helplessness I felt that day, wondering if my son would ever be able to eat what he wanted. Would he ever be able to enjoy certain types of foods just like everyone else? Likewise, I'll never forget the paralyzing fear I felt realizing that I was solely responsible for keeping my son safe and alive. After a few weepy minutes, I dug in and got to work doing the only thing I could do—make the best of an intimidating situation. I started my lonely journey with a trip to the grocery store, bearing a list of ingredients to avoid. After weeks, months, and years of trial and error, I managed to develop some simply wonderful recipes that please the whole family.

Eating out with food allergies is difficult, and I generally avoid it. There's simply no security in it. As a mom of a child with multiple food allergies, I've learned the risk and worry aren't worth it. I decided early on that cooking and baking at home is the best and safest option. And here's the best part: baking with your children is a fantastic way to bring your family together. My kids already know their way around the kitchen, and they use their imaginations to make up their own recipes. This is especially important for John, as he'll need to learn to cook for himself once he's all grown up. Unless a cure is found for food allergies, he'll have to fend for himself in college and beyond.

Whenever another mom tells me she failed to make a recipe well, I always respond that she didn't fail the recipe—the recipe failed her. A disappointing result is enough to shake the confidence of any home baker. A mom who bakes allergen-free can't afford to have her confidence shaken. She can't just go out to the grocery store and pick up another birthday cake if her recipe doesn't turn out right.

Here's a little secret about baking with food allergies: it isn't that big of a deal. It just means making simple adjustments to how you bake by using safe, allergen-free ingredients. In developing the recipes for this book, I made sure to use good-quality ingredients that are widely available and affordable. The recipes are simple and easy to follow, yet full of home-baked goodness that will rival any traditional recipe containing dairy, eggs, and/or nuts.

There are several food-allergy cookbooks on the market that dutifully explain the mechanics of allergen-free cooking and baking, and they are filled with hundreds of recipes that are free of common allergens. *The Food Allergy Mama's Baking Book: Great Dairy, Egg, and Nut-Free Treats for the Whole Family* isn't that kind of cookbook. *The Food Allergy Mama's Baking Book* is intended to provide busy moms of food-allergic children with the very best dairy, egg, peanut, and tree nut-free baking recipes. Each recipe is carefully written for the home baker who wants simple recipes that work well and taste delicious.

I hope you enjoy this book as much as I have enjoyed writing it. It has meant the world to me to see my son enjoy wonderful desserts he'd never be able to have elsewhere, right here in my own kitchen. Shouldn't every kid have his cake, and eat it too?

PART ONE

The Food Allergy Mama's Tips and Advice

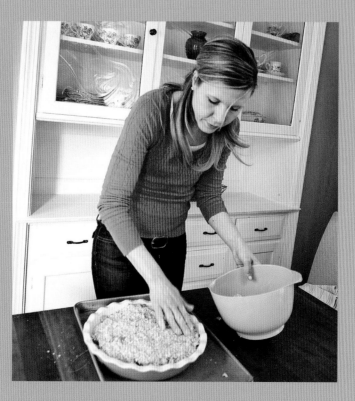

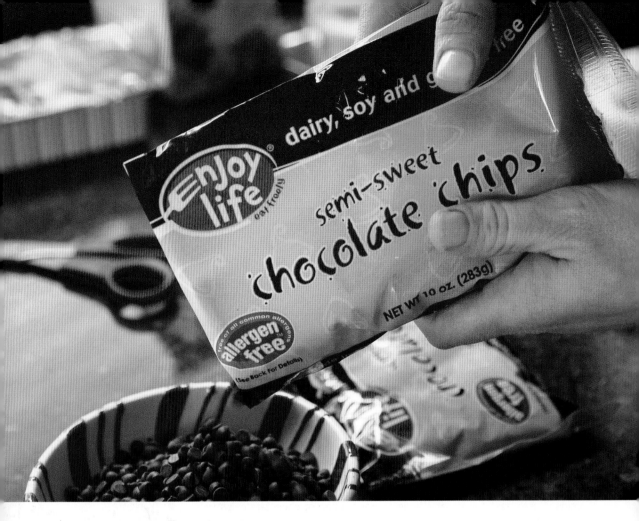

Top Dairy, Egg, and Nut-Free Ingredients

As a mother of four young children, my daily life is far too hectic to spend all day shopping for exotic ingredients. Besides, the cost to feed those four little mouths increases every year (especially since they keep getting bigger!), so I'm not about to spend a lot of money on egg substitutes and fancy organic products. I pick and choose where I spend my money. Here's a list of favorite ingredients I use in all my recipes:

NIELSEN-MASSEY PURE VANILLA EXTRACT. Nope, this isn't necessarily inexpensive and easy to find in your local supermarket, but the quality can't be matched. Don't go cheap with your vanilla. Always make sure you get the good stuff. You can find it at Williams-Sonoma and Whole Foods Markets.

GOLD MEDAL UNBLEACHED ALL-PURPOSE FLOUR. I prefer using the unbleached version, because it's spared the additional chemical processing of bleached flour. You can find it at your local grocery store.

DAIRY-FREE SHORTENING. If plain Crisco was good enough for James Beard, it's good enough for me. I bake a lot, so I always want ingredients I can pick up at the grocery store. I have also used Earth Balance shortening and Spectrum Organic shortening with success.

FLEISCHMANN'S UNSALTED MARGARINE. I always get great results from my traditional recipes when I use dairy-free margarine in place of butter. The unsalted version is dairy free and contains soy. Earth Balance Buttery Sticks could also be used in recipes that call for dairy-free margarine.

CRISCO BAKING SPRAY WITH FLOUR. This stuff is pure magic—no more mess from greasing and flouring pans! I use it to spray every cake and muffin pan, and even my hot griddle when I make pancakes. Important note: Only use the plain version with flour, and never buy butter-flavored sprays, as they often contain milk products.

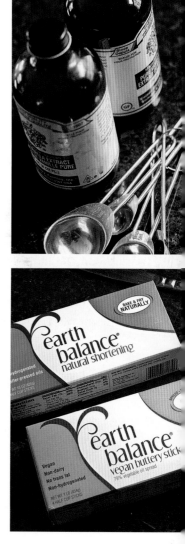

DAIRY, EGG, AND NUT-FREE CHOCOLATE CHIPS. In the world of dairy-, egg-, and nut-free baking, there are only two commercial brands I turn to for chips: Divvies and Enjoy Life. I searched high and low for a totally safe chocolate chip and was always stopped in my tracks by that "shared equipment" disclaimer. Either the dairy-free chips I found were produced in facilities that also produced nut-containing products, or the chips from nut-free facilities contained dairy. Divvies is a wonderful company that is dedicated to providing dairy-, egg-, and nut-free sweet treats, including cookies, caramel corn, and candy. The Sandler family founded the company to meet the needs of their son, who suffers from life-threatening food allergies, so it is very comforting to know that they put as much care into making a safe, allergen-free product as I would. Their chocolate chips are larger and similar in size to traditional chips. Customers can order a large (5–pound) bag of chocolate chips from the Divvies Website. Enjoy Life is another company that is allergen aware. It has extremely strict supplier agreements and batch tests every product that comes out of its dedicated facility for trace allergens. Their chocolate chips are miniature in size, and are available at Whole Foods stores.

UNSWEETENED APPLESAUCE. You'll notice I use a lot of applesauce in my recipes because it gives just the right amount of moisture to cookies and muffins. Only use unsweetened applesauce in your recipes, because the sugary versions will add too much sweetness to your baked goods.

VINEGAR. Plain white vinegar is a great egg replacer and can turn ordinary soy milk into buttermilk (see page 19).

SILKEN TOFU. Tofu is one of my favorite choices for an egg replacer when my baked goods need more density. I prefer Nasoya brand silken tofu.

TOFUTTI DAIRY-FREE SOUR CREAM AND CREAM CHEESE. For recipes with cream cheese as a main ingredient, such as cheesecake and key lime pie, I use Tofutti. It tastes great and has a rich, thick consistency.

Top Baking Hints

MAKE SURE YOUR OVEN IS ALWAYS PROPERLY PREHEATED, AND GET AN OVEN THERMOMETER. I've given general time recommendations in the book, because some ovens are hotter than others. Buy an oven thermometer so you'll know where your oven's hot spots are.

MEASURE FLOUR AND OTHER DRY INGREDIENTS PROPERLY. Baking is a science, so it isn't wise to just wing it, throwing a little of this and a little of that into your recipes. Measure flour and other dry ingredients by spooning them into measuring cups and leveling them with a straight edge (the reverse side of a spoon works fine). Doing so ensures you are getting the most accurate measurement possible. The exception to this rule is brown sugar, which is always pressed and packed into a measuring cup.

ALWAYS USE A CLEAR GLASS LIQUID MEASURING CUP FOR LIQUIDS. Pour the amount needed into the measuring cup, and bend down to carefully check that the liquid reaches the proper level and the measurement is exact.

NEVER MEASURE INGREDIENTS OVER YOUR MIXING BOWL. The last thing you'll want to do is pour too much salt (or anything else, for that matter) into a measuring spoon and have it overflow into your bowl of measured ingredients.

SCRAPE THE BOWL OFTEN AS YOU MIX INGREDIENTS. I've made the mistake of not scraping the bowl regularly as I blend ingredients together, only to find clumps of ingredients at the bottom that weren't properly incorporated.

USE A TIMER. Don't try to remember when the cookies should come out of the oven. Let the timer remind you instead.

USE GOOD-QUALITY EQUIPMENT. Invest in good equipment and you'll bake with consistent results. Heavy aluminum baking sheets, heavy-duty mixers, good measuring cups, cherry pitters, and other kitchen essentials will last practically forever if you invest in the good stuff the first time around.

WEAR AN APRON. I know this isn't really equipment, but my aprons are about as important as anything else I use in the kitchen. Invariably, you'll end up wearing a lot of flour, vanilla, vinegar, and who knows what else as you put these recipes together. Protect yourself and your cute clothes.

KNOW YOUR BAKING SHEETS AND THEIR SIZES. Shiny aluminum baking sheets produce the most even results. Baking a cake in a 15×10-inch jelly-roll pan will produce a different result than baking in a 13×9-inch cake pan. Use the right pan for the recipe.

READ YOUR RECIPES THOROUGHLY BEFORE YOU BEGIN. Make sure you have all the necessary ingredients and equipment. The last thing you want to happen is to get started and realize halfway through that you don't have a key ingredient.

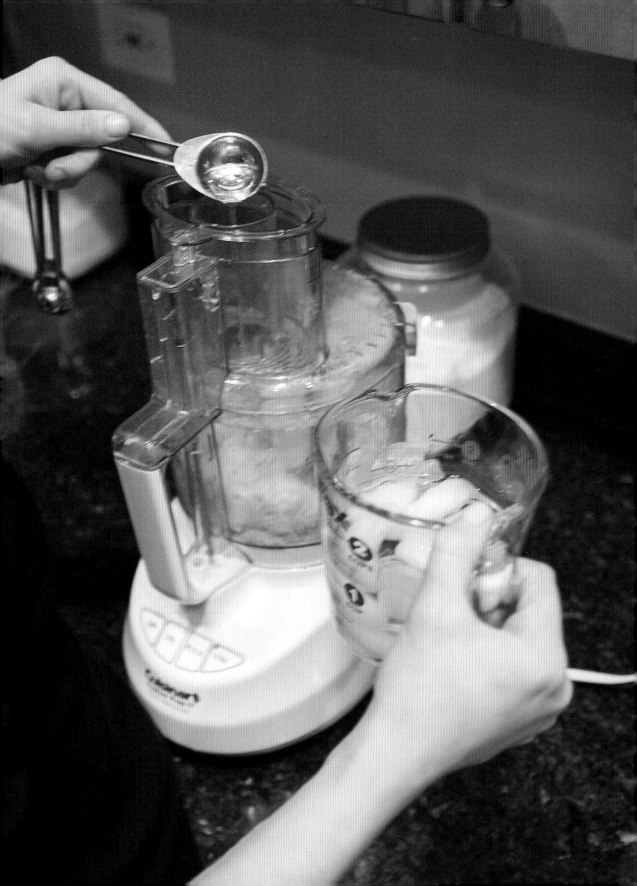

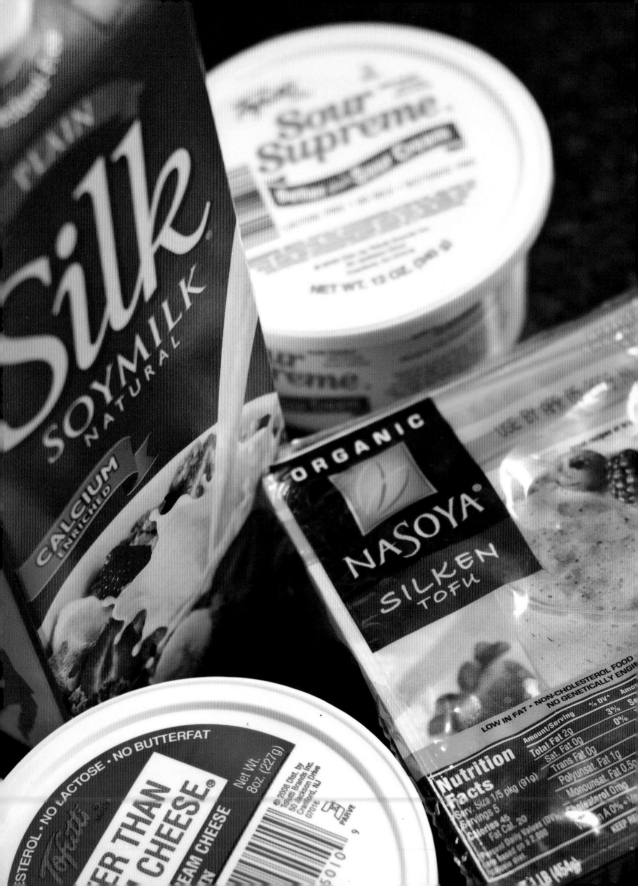

Top Dairy Substitutes

SILK BRAND PLAIN SOY MILK. This is the milk we drink at our house, so that's what I use for baking. Use 1 cup of soy milk for every cup of dairy milk.

DAIRY-FREE BUTTERMILK. Make your own cup of dairy-free buttermilk by placing 1 tablespoon plain white vinegar or 1 tablespoon fresh lemon juice into a measuring cup and adding soy milk until you reach a 1-cup measure. Let the mixture sit 5 to 10 minutes before using.

DAIRY-FREE MARGARINE AND SHORTENING. Use the same measurements as you would for dairy butter.

DAIRY-FREE SOUR CREAM AND CREAM CHEESE. Substitute Tofutti's delicious tofu-based products for recipes that call for sour cream or cream cheese.

DAIRY-FREE HEAVY CREAM. Make your own heavy cream by simply puréeing silken tofu in a blender. Use the same amount, cup for cup, you would of real cream.

Top Egg and Nut Substitutes

UNSWEETENED APPLESAUCE. Replace each egg with ¼ cup unsweetened applesauce.

MASHED BANANA. Replace each egg with ¼ cup mashed banana.

SILKEN TOFU. Replace each egg with ¼ cup tofu.

WATER. Replace each egg with 1 tablespoon water.

FLAX MEAL. Replace each egg with 1 tablespoon flax meal and 3 tablespoons hot water; let stand 5 minutes, until thickened.

SOY NUT BUTTER. Soy nut butter is the only peanut/tree-nut substitute I use in my baking. I especially like the I.M. Healthy brand, which you can easily find in your local supermarket or Whole Foods stores.

Favorite Baking Tools

There are a few tools and pans I turn to time and again. I don't believe in fancy equipment or hot new gadgets, but I do believe in a few tools that will make your baking life easier.

PARCHMENT PAPER. These little sheets of paper will work magic for your baked goods. Never again will you have burnt cookie bottoms.

COOKIE SCOOPER. I use this little gadget to scoop perfectly proportioned pieces of cookie dough onto my baking sheets. I also use it to place pancake batter on a hot griddle.

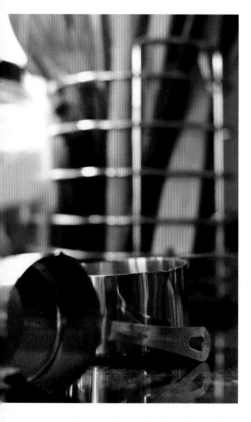

KITCHEN AID STAND MIXER. I especially love the Kitchen Aid's dough hook attachment, because it makes mixing ingredients for homemade bread and pizza dough super easy.

SEVERAL LIQUID MEASURING CUPS WITH 4- AND 2-CUP CAPACITIES. I use liquid measuring cups all the time to measure out water, soy milk, buttermilk, and puréed tofu. It's a good idea to have plenty of clean, dry cups on hand.

RASP ZESTER. It's a breeze to grate lemon zest with one of these. I recommend Microplane brand zesters; they are reasonably priced and of superior quality.

PYREX 13×9-INCH, 9-INCH SQUARE, AND 9-INCH ROUND GLASS BAKING DISHES. I still have my mother's 13×9-inch Pyrex baking dish, and I use my 9-inch square dish for brownies, cobblers, and crisps. Pyrex glass dishes produce the most consistent results.

JUICE REAMER. I like to use a lot of citrus juice and zest in my recipes to brighten the flavors. This inexpensive little gadget is the fastest way to juice a citrus fruit. Use its pointed end to remove the seeds prior to juicing.

FOOD PROCESSOR. Making pie dough is a breeze in the food processor. See recipe on page 134.

PYREX DIGITAL PROBE OVEN THERMOMETER AND TIMER. I use timers every time I bake. I like the Pyrex brand product best, because the probe comes in handy when I need to check water temperatures for my yeast bread recipes.

MIXING BOWLS IN A VARIETY OF SIZES. I use 2- and 4-quart bowls most frequently, but it is always good to have a wide range of bowls and sizes. They all serve different purposes.

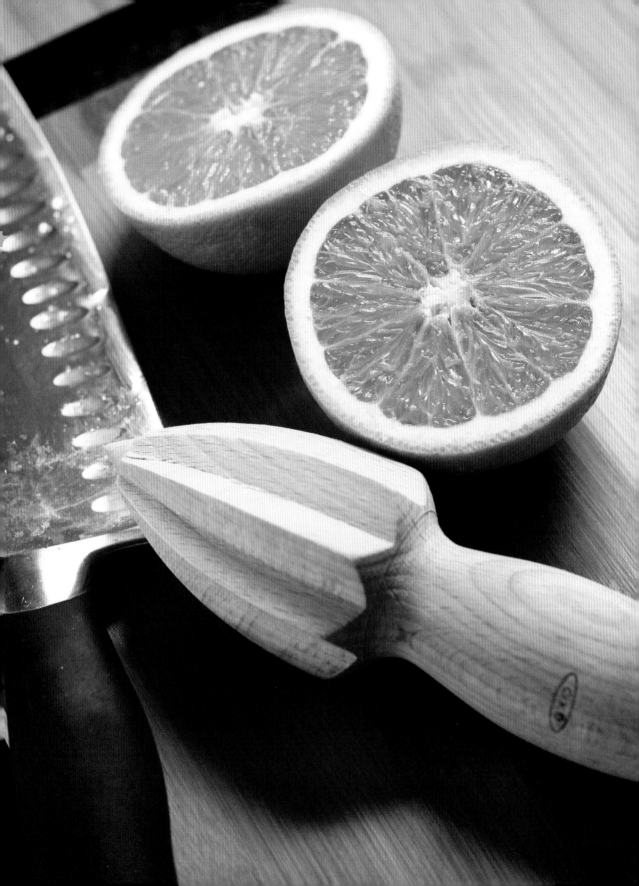

Tips for Reading Product Labels

For food labeling information, I always consult the Food Allergy and Anaphylaxis Network (FAAN) at www.foodallergy.org. FAAN is the go-to resource for absolutely anyone, whether you have just been diagnosed or have been coping with food allergies for years. FAAN's site is dedicated to providing up-to-date and thorough information on the eight major allergens: milk, eggs, peanuts, tree nuts, fish, shellfish, soy, and wheat. Visit it to review, download, or print useful information about food processing and ingredients, chef's cards, and product recall alerts.

The aim of the U.S. Food Allergen Labeling and Consumer Protection Act, which took effect January 1, 2006, was to make it easy for even young children to be able to read clear, standardized food labels so they would not accidentally consume potentially hazardous allergens. When I first learned about the law, I thought, "Great! Now I won't have to read every label with a magnifying glass." Unfortunately, my son suffered a couple of allergic reactions to mislabeled products before I learned my lesson. You must still carefully read every ingredient. Skipping to the section of the label that starts with "Contains" and lists known allergens may mean skipping over some potentially harmful substances. Even if you are very careful, you still aren't guaranteed full disclosure by food manufacturers: many products have been recalled in years past for not declaring potential allergens.

Since products made with milk, eggs, peanuts, and tree nuts often go by other names in ingredient lists, here is a helpful list of ingredient names to avoid:

Milk

Artificial butter flavor

Butter (butter fat, butter oil, and buttermilk)

Casein

Caseinates (ammonium, calcium, magnesium, and potassium)

Cheese

Cottage cheese

Cream

Curds

Custard

Half-and-half

High-protein flour

Hydrolysates (casein, milk protein, whey, and whey protein)

Lactalbumin and lactalbumin phosphate

Lactoglobulin

Lactose

Malted, condensed, evaporated, dry, whole,

low-fat, nonfat, skimmed, and goat milk

Margarine (Fleischmann's Unsalted Margarine is dairy free—it contains only soy)

Milk derivative, milk protein, and milk solids

Nougat

Pudding

Rennet casein

Some flavorings, such as caramel, cream, coconut cream, and chocolate

Sour cream

Whey (delactosed, demineralized, and protein concentrate)

Yogurt

Eggs

Albumin

Egg lecithin

Egg substitutes

Egg white, egg yolk, dried egg, and powdered egg

Eggnot

Globulin

Livetin

Mayonnaise

Meringue

Ovalbumin

Ovomucin

Ovomucoid

Ovovitellin

Peanuts

Candy

Chocolate

Cold-pressed peanut oil

Ground nuts

Marzipan

Most bakery treats

Mixed nuts

Nougat

Nu nuts

Peanut butter

Peanut flour

Tree Nuts

Almond paste

Almonds

Brazil nuts

Cashews

Chestnuts

Filberts

Hazelnuts

Hickory nuts

Macadamia nuts

Marzipan

Nougat

Nu nuts

Nut butters

Nut meal

Nut oil

Nut paste

Pecans

Pine nuts

Pistachios

Walnuts

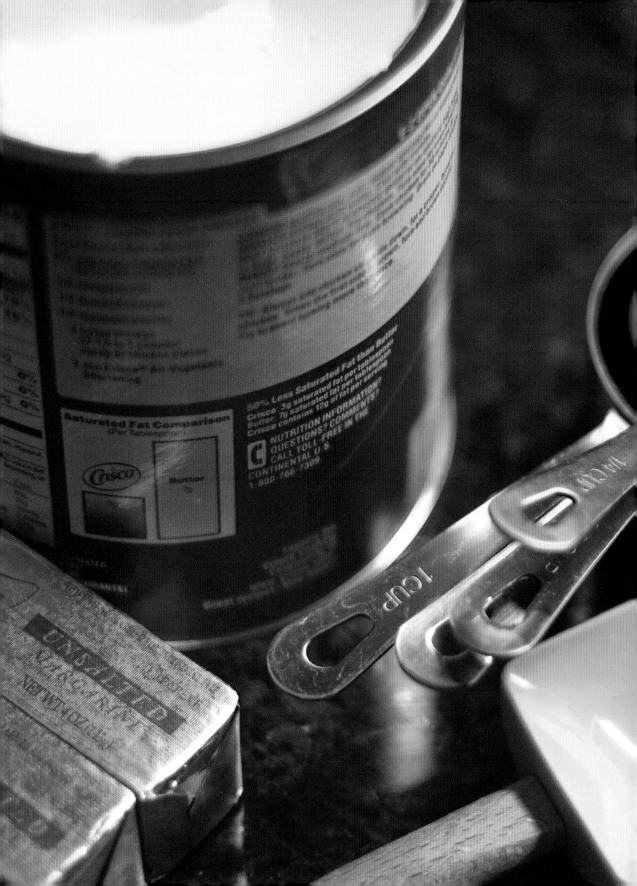

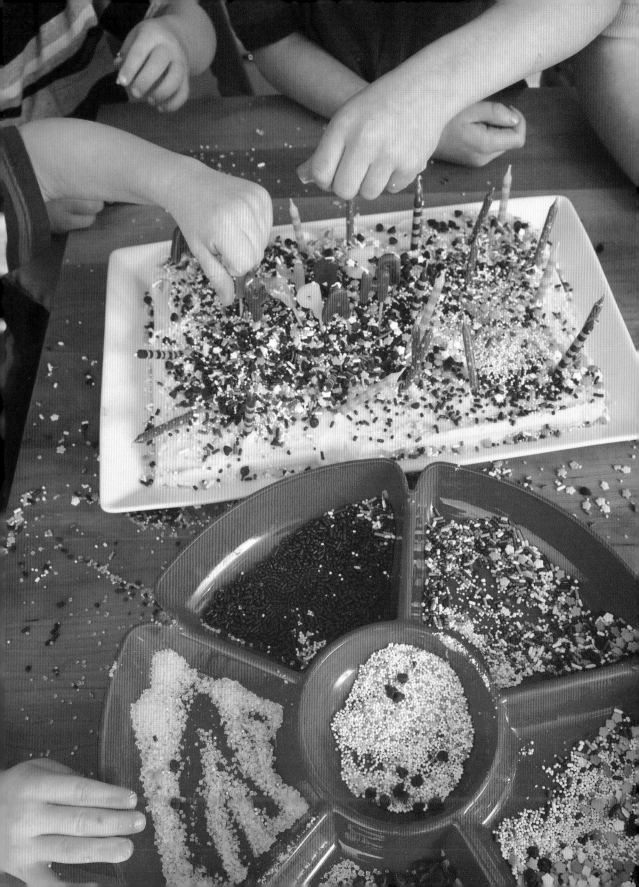

Tips for Birthday and Classroom Parties

Birthday and classroom parties are a part of every child's life. For the food-allergic child (and his or her parents), it can be a source of great anxiety—but it doesn't have to be if you arrive prepared. Here are some tips to help you get through any celebration.

Birthday Parties

CALL THE HOST AS SOON AS YOU GET THE INVITATION. Tell the party host about your child's food allergies. Find out what food will be served and determine if anything will be suitable for your child to eat. Discuss the severity of your child's allergies and recommend that surface areas be wiped down before and after eating. Keep wet wipes or a hand sanitizer at the tables so all the children will be able to clean their hands.

ALWAYS SEND A SEPARATE SNACK AND TREAT WITH YOUR CHILD. Many parents want to safely accommodate your child's allergies and will ask what they can do to help him or her feel included. Healthy treats, such as fresh fruit kabobs, pretzels, and crackers, are great choices. However, when it comes to the birthday cake, be prepared to send a separate treat. Make a batch of my Chocolate or Vanilla Cupcakes (see pages 111 and 112), and freeze the extras for another party down the road. You can purchase Cup-a-Cake plastic cupcake holders (www.cupacake.com) that are perfect for transporting single-serve cupcakes and muffins. Williams-Sonoma carries this brand as well.

SHOW UP EARLY. Remind the host about your child's food allergies, and bring along a rescue medicine kit with dual epinephrine autoinjectors (EpiPens), antihistamines, and, if needed, an asthma inhaler. Place a complete copy of your child's Food Allergy Action Plan (downloadable atwww.foodallergy.org/actionplan.pdf) inside the kit. Explain to the party host what symptoms he or she should look for if an allergen is accidentally ingested and show the host how to use an EpiPen. If you plan to leave your child at the party, give the host your emergency contact information and keep your phone close by.

REMIND THE HOST TO ALWAYS TAKE ACTION, EVEN IF HE OR SHE IS IN DOUBT ABOUT WHETHER YOUR CHILD IS SUFFERING FROM AN ALLERGIC REACTION. Even a food-allergic child's own parent is sometimes afraid to administer an EpiPen the first time. Reassure the host that epinephrine won't harm your child, but it could save his or her life. If a reaction is suspected, the host should quickly follow the guidelines in the Food Allergy Action Plan.

RELAX AND REMIND YOUR CHILD TO HAVE FUN. Yes, food is a part of the party experience, but it isn't everything. Try to take the emphasis off the food and remind your child to have fun playing the games and taking part in the celebration. The less anxious you are, the less anxious your child will be.

Classroom Parties

At least until your child enters middle school, classroom parties will probably be a part of his or her life. Each school district has its own policy on how to handle birthday and holiday celebrations in the classroom. Children with food allergies can be considered disabled under Section 504 of the

Rehabilitation Act and the Americans with Disabilities Act (ADA). Section 504 requires schools to provide "free, appropriate education" regardless of any condition—physical, mental, or emotional—that could interfere with a student's ability to receive an education in a public-school classroom. The endangerment of a child's personal safety if hazardous food allergens are present in a classroom falls under this umbrella.

Since there is still a lack of understanding about the severity of food allergies—and young children cannot be their own advocates—I have always made sure to have a 504 Plan on file at

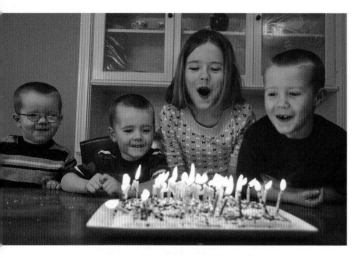

my child's school. A 504 Plan legally binds your child's school to provide appropriate care within its classrooms and keep him or her safe.

However, this doesn't mean he or she is protected if well-meaning parents bring in unsafe treats to share during classroom celebrations. Some school districts have adopted a "treat-free" policy prohibiting treats and other food in class. Some parents who aren't familiar with the severity of food allergies may become upset because they can't bring in special treats to share. Foods containing potentially hazardous allergens can trigger life-threatening allergic reactions, but they also ultimately make food-allergic children feel excluded. These are difficult concepts for young children to grasp, so it's important to be your child's advocate at all times. Educating other parents and the school's staff is the only way to get past these issues and keep your child safe. Here are some helpful tips when dealing with treats in your child's classroom.

HAVE A 504 PLAN ON FILE AT YOUR CHILD'S SCHOOL. In order to have a 504 Plan, your child's food allergy condition must "substantially limit one or more of life's activities." Meet with staff from your child's school to discuss his or her eligibility, which is determined by the severity of the food allergy and your child's ability to self-advocate.

MEET WITH YOUR CHILD'S TEACHER BEFORE THE START OF THE SCHOOL YEAR. Discuss your child's allergy, and work together to create a game plan for birthday celebrations and holiday parties. If birthdays are celebrated in the classroom, ask your child's teacher to adopt a nonfood celebration policy. Instead of sending cupcakes, cookies, and candy to school, parents could instead send in fun trinkets, such as stickers, pencils, games, or books, or visit the classroom to read a story. For holiday parties, ask parents to bring in festive healthy snacks, such as fresh fruit, sliced veggies, etc.

ASK YOUR CHILD'S TEACHER TO SEND OUT A LETTER ABOUT FOOD ALLERGIES AT THE BEGINNING OF THE YEAR. Parents who don't have children with food allergies sometimes just aren't aware of how dangerous food allergies can be. A letter that details the specific food allergies of children in the classroom, what snacks are acceptable, and the school's policy about food celebrations will help avoid confrontations and confusion down the road.

Top Questions about Food Allergies

There is no cure for food allergies. Over 12 million Americans suffer from this potentially fatal disease, and nearly 150 to 200 people die from anaphylactic shock every year. Living with food allergies isn't a choice: it is a real disability that food-allergic individuals have to live with every single day.

WHAT IS A FOOD ALLERGY? It is the body's immune response to food it believes to be harmful. When food-allergic individuals eat a harmful food, their bodies create specific antibodies to it. Their bodies react to the presence of the food by sending out huge amounts of chemicals to fight it. This flood of chemicals triggers a variety of symptoms, which could possibly include hives, itching, gastrointestinal distress, and cardiovascular and respiratory issues. In the most severe cases, anaphylactic shock will occur.

WHAT IS ANAPHYLACTIC SHOCK? It is the most serious of allergic reactions, which, if left untreated, can quickly lead to death. The patient's blood pressure drops dramatically and the airway constricts until he or she cannot breathe.

WHAT ARE THE SYMPTOMS OF ANAPHYLACTIC REACTIONS? Symptoms may begin with hives, itching, or tingling in the mouth and can rapidly progress to vomiting, diarrhea, labored breathing, excessive coughing, a sudden drop in blood pressure, and loss of consciousness.

HOW DO YOU TREAT THESE TYPES OF ALLERGIC REACTIONS? Food-allergic individuals should have a rescue medicine kit with them at all times. The kit should include two epinephrine autoinjectors (autoinjectors are always sold in packages of two, so you have a backup in case one injector fails), an antihistamine, and an asthma inhaler, if needed.

WHAT IS THE BEST TREATMENT PLAN? The safest plan is to strictly avoid any food the person is allergic to.

PART TWO

The Recipes

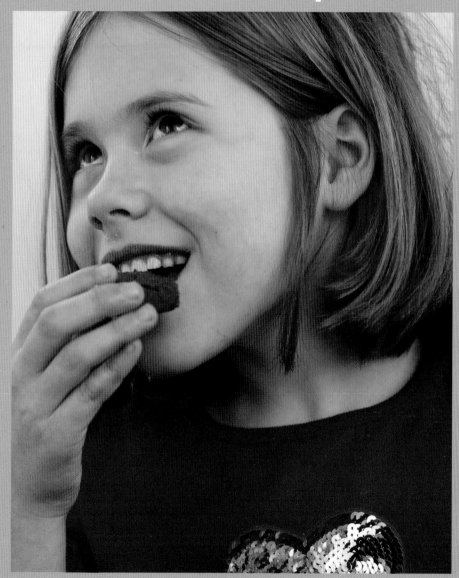

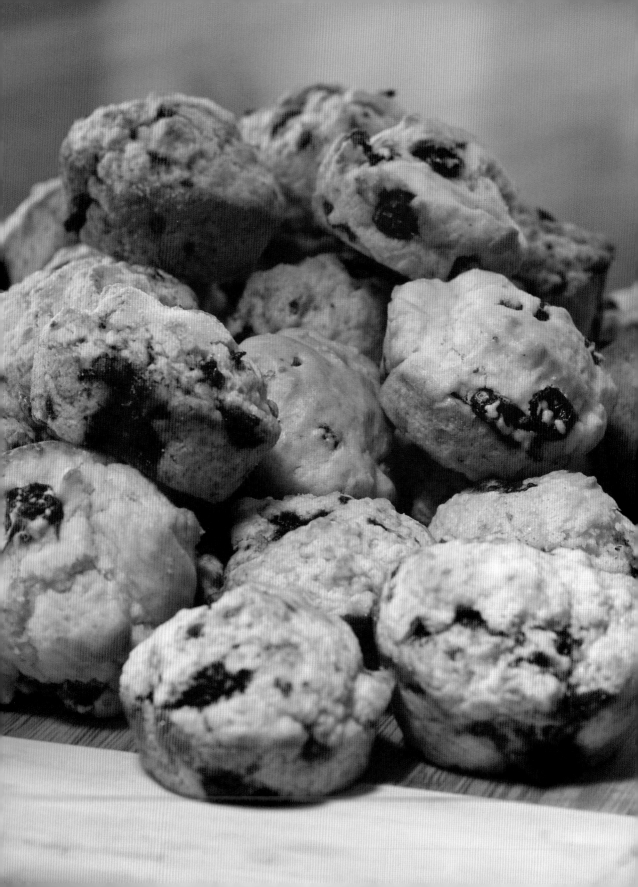

THE FOOD ALLERGY MAMA'S
Quick Breads, Muffins, and More

When I want to bake something sweet with my children but don't have a lot of time, I often turn to my quick-bread and muffin recipes. They are simple to make and require few ingredients. Mixing the batter is a breeze, either with or without a stand mixer. These recipes are perfect to make with your children: children love to eat simple, home-baked goods as much they love to make them.

In this chapter, there are also great recipes for pancakes, doughnuts, and waffles—foods that are usually a big taboo for those with food allergies. Eating these types of foods at restaurants or bakeries is often out of the question, but my versions of these items are so good, you won't be able to tell they're completely dairy, egg, and nut-free. These are dishes you and your family can turn to again and again.

The best part about making these recipes is that most of them can be frozen after cooling and reheated and served later. Even the pancakes and waffles freeze beautifully, which is great when you want to serve your kids a warm breakfast but are short on time.

Cinnamon Bread

This bread has a delicious layer of cinnamon crunch on top. My family usually devours this loaf as soon as it comes out of the oven.

YIELD: 1 LOAF

Bread

¼ cup dairy-free shortening (see page 15)

¾ cup granulated sugar

2 tablespoons water

2 cups unbleached all-purpose flour

1 tablespoon baking powder

1½ teaspoons ground cinnamon

¾ teaspoon salt

1 cup soy or rice milk

Topping

2 teaspoons ground cinnamon

½ cup granulated sugar

2 teaspoons melted dairy-free margarine

Preheat oven to 375°F, and spray a 9×5×3-inch loaf pan with dairy-free baking spray.

In the bowl of a stand mixer fitted with the paddle attachment, cream together the shortening and ¾ cup sugar thoroughly, adding the water as the mixer runs. Beat until fluffy.

In a separate mixing bowl, sift together the remaining dry ingredients: flour, baking powder, cinnamon, and salt. Add the dry mixture to the shortening mixture, alternating it with the soy milk.

In a separate bowl, mix together the 2 teaspoons cinnamon, the ½ cup sugar, and the margarine to make the topping.

Pour the batter into the prepared loaf pan. Sprinkle the batter with the topping mixture. Bake for 45 minutes, or until an inserted cake tester comes out clean and the topping is crusty brown. Cool 10 minutes before slicing.

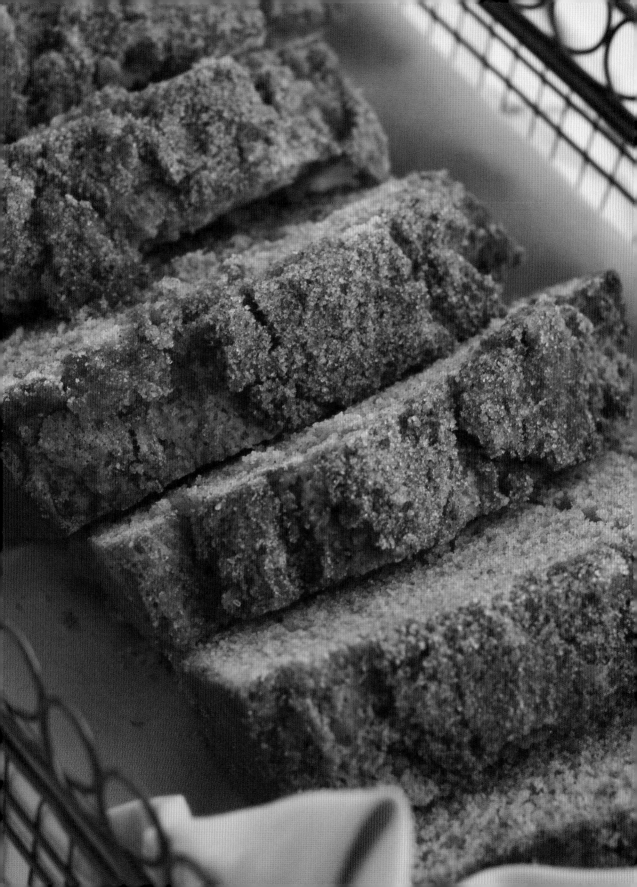

Cinnamon–Raisin Bread

Sure, there are some allergen-free cinnamon raisin breads at the store, but this is so much fresher. Why not make your own?

YIELD: 1 LOAF

2 tablespoons water

1¾ cups dairy-free buttermilk (2 cups soy or rice milk mixed with 2 tablespoons white vinegar; let it sit for 5–10 minutes)

3 cups unbleached all-purpose flour

⅔ cup granulated sugar

3 teaspoons baking powder

2 teaspoons ground cinnamon

1 teaspoon baking soda

1 teaspoon salt

2 tablespoons dairy-free margarine, melted

1¾ cups raisins

Preheat oven to 350°F, and spray a 9×5×3-inch loaf pan with dairy-free baking spray.

In a small bowl, mix together the water and buttermilk with a small whisk. Set aside. In a large bowl, combine the flour, sugar, baking powder, cinnamon, baking soda, and salt with a wire whisk. Fold in the buttermilk mixture and melted margarine using a rubber spatula. Add the raisins and stir well.

Pour the batter into a prepared loaf pan, and bake for 55 to 60 minutes, or until an inserted cake tester comes out clean.

Cool completely before slicing.

Strawberry Bread

I love the combination of strawberries and oranges. The recipe calls for frozen strawberries, which is great if you want to make this bread year-round.

YIELD: 1 LOAF

1½ cups frozen strawberries

½ cup vegetable oil

3 tablespoons water

½ cup unsweetened applesauce

2 teaspoons freshly squeezed orange juice

2 teaspoons grated orange zest

2½ cups unbleached all-purpose flour

1 cup granulated sugar

1½ teaspoons ground cinnamon

¾ teaspoon baking soda

¼ teaspoon salt

Preheat oven to 350°F, and spray a 9×5×3-inch loaf pan with dairy-free baking spray.

In a blender, purée the strawberries, oil, water, applesauce, orange juice, and orange zest until smooth.

In a medium bowl, combine the flour, sugar, cinnamon, baking soda, and salt with a wire whisk. Make a well in the middle of the flour mixture, and pour the strawberry purée into the well. Stir with a rubber spatula until just combined.

Pour into the prepared pan, and bake for 50 to 60 minutes, or until an inserted cake tester comes out clean.

Cool completely before slicing.

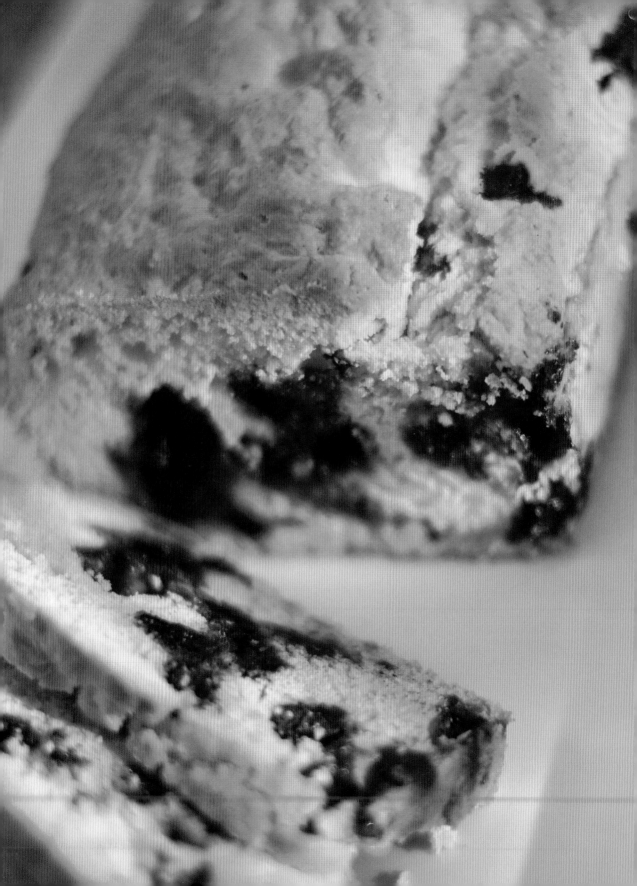

Pumpkin Bread

I love this bread; it is one of my favorites to make during the fall season. This recipe makes two loaves, which makes it perfect to share with neighbors and friends. It also freezes well.

YIELD: 2 LOAVES

⅔ cup dairy-free shortening (see page 15)

2½ cups granulated sugar

4 tablespoons water

1 (15-ounce) can puréed pumpkin (not pumpkin pie filling)

¼ cup orange juice

3 cups unbleached all-purpose flour

2 teaspoons baking soda

1 teaspoon baking powder

1 teaspoon ground cinnamon

½ teaspoon salt

½ teaspoon nutmeg

Preheat oven to 350°F, and spray two 8-inch loaf pans with dairy-free baking spray.

In the bowl of a stand mixer fitted with the paddle attachment, cream together the shortening and sugar. Add the water, pumpkin, and orange juice, and mix well.

In a medium bowl, combine the flour, baking soda, baking powder, cinnamon, salt, and nutmeg with a wire whisk. Add this dry mixture to the shortening mixture, and combine thoroughly. Pour into the prepared loaf pans, and bake for 50 to 60 minutes, or until an inserted cake tester comes out clean.

Cool completely before serving.

Freezing Tip: To freeze bread for later, wrap tightly in plastic wrap and then in aluminum foil. Label with name and date, and freeze for up to 2 months.

Zucchini Bread

I've tried and tested lots of zucchini recipes, but most were too heavy, oily, and sugary for my taste. I like the natural flavor of the zucchini to come out. This zucchini bread has half the oil of many other recipes, but you don't miss a thing. An unexpected bonus is the lightly crisped crust.

YIELD: 2 LOAVES

4 tablespoons water

½ cup vegetable oil

½ cup unsweetened applesauce

2 cups granulated sugar

1 teaspoon vanilla extract

2 cups grated, unpeeled zucchini

4 cups unbleached all-purpose flour

3½ teaspoons ground cinnamon

2 teaspoons baking soda

1½ teaspoons baking powder

1 teaspoon salt

Preheat oven to 350°F, and spray two 8-inch loaf pans with dairy-free baking spray.

In the bowl of a stand mixer fitted with the paddle attachment, combine the water, vegetable oil, applesauce, sugar, and vanilla. Stir in the zucchini and mix well.

In a medium bowl, combine the flour, cinnamon, baking soda, baking powder, and salt with a wire whisk. Stir the dry ingredients into the zucchini mixture until just combined. Pour into the prepared pans, and bake for 50 to 60 minutes, or until an inserted cake tester comes out clean.

Cool completely before slicing.

Banana Bread

Make sure your bananas are nicely browned, because very ripe bananas produce the best breads. Make one for now, and freeze the other for later.

YIELD: 2 LOAVES

½ cup dairy-free margarine

1⅓ cups granulated sugar

1½ cups mashed ripe banana

3 tablespoons water

2¾ cups unbleached all-purpose flour

2½ teaspoons baking powder

½ teaspoon salt

¾ cup dairy-free buttermilk (1 cup soy or rice milk mixed with 1 tablespoons white vinegar; let it sit for 5–10 minutes)

Preheat oven to 350°F, and spray two 8-inch baking pans with dairy-free baking spray.

In the bowl of a stand mixer fitted with the paddle attachment, combine the margarine, sugar, banana, and water. In a medium bowl, combine the flour, baking powder, and salt with a wire whisk.

Alternate adding the flour mixture and the buttermilk to the margarine–banana mixture, starting and ending with the flour mixture. Pour into the prepared pans, and bake for 50 to 60 minutes, or until an inserted cake tester comes clean.

Cool completely before slicing.

Blueberry Bread

This is a perfect bread to serve for breakfast; it bursts with blueberries and has a nice hint of orange in it.

YIELD: 1 LOAF

½ cup dairy-free margarine, melted

3 tablespoons water

½ cup soy or rice milk

2 tablespoons grated orange zest

⅔ cup orange juice

3 cups unbleached all-purpose flour

¾ cup granulated sugar

1 tablespoon baking powder

¾ teaspoon salt

¼ teaspoon baking soda

1 cup blueberries, fresh or frozen

Preheat oven to 350°F, and spray a 9×5×3-inch loaf pan with dairy-free baking spray.

In the bowl of a stand mixer fitted with the paddle attachment, combine the melted margarine, water, soy milk, orange zest, and orange juice until thoroughly combined. In a medium bowl, combine the flour, sugar, baking powder, salt, and baking soda with a wire whisk. Add the dry mixture to the margarine mixture, and stir with a rubber spatula until just combined. Fold in the blueberries.

Pour the batter into a prepared loaf pan, and bake for 55 to 60 minutes, or until the top is golden brown. Cool completely before slicing.

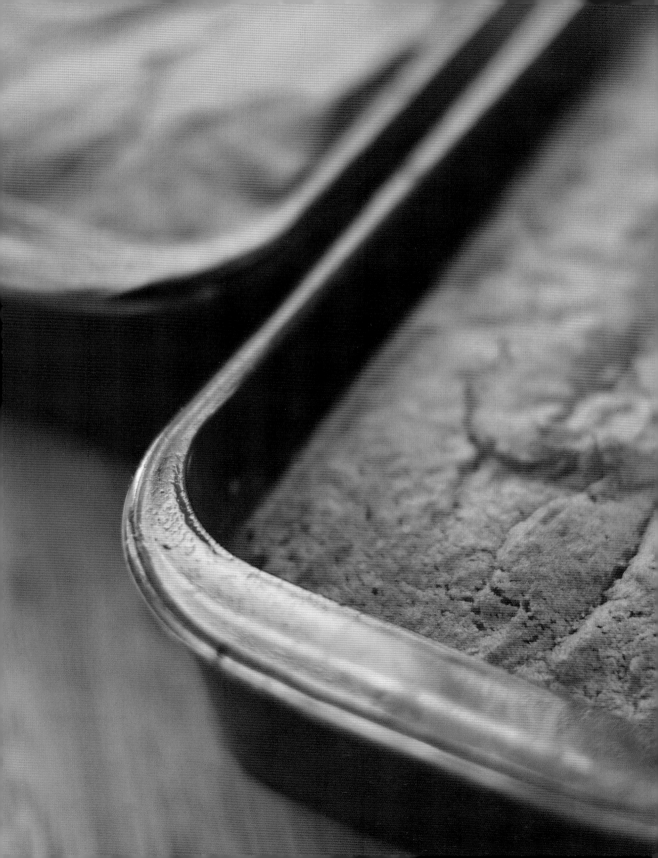

Cranberry Bread

This was a popular recipe on my blog at www.foodallergymama.com. The bread itself resembles a pound cake peppered with bright red cranberries. It is perfect to serve during the holiday season.

YIELD: 2 LOAVES

1 cup plus 2 tablespoons water

½ cup dairy-free margarine, melted

2 cups orange juice

Grated zest of 1 orange

5 cups unbleached all-purpose flour

2½ cups granulated sugar

3 teaspoons baking powder

1 teaspoon baking soda

1½ teaspoons salt

1 cup whole cranberries, fresh or frozen

Preheat oven to 325°F, and spray two 9-inch loaf pans with dairy-free baking spray.

In the bowl of a stand mixer fitted with the paddle attachment, combine the water, melted margarine, orange juice, and orange zest. In a medium bowl, combine the flour, sugar, baking powder, baking soda, and salt with a wire whisk.

Make a well in the center of the dry ingredients, and pour the wet mixture into the well. Stir just until moist. Fold in the cranberries, and pour the batter into the prepared pans. Bake for 50 to 60 minutes, or until an inserted cake tester comes out clean.

Cool completely before slicing.

Waffles

Kids with food allergies can't eat just any frozen waffles from the grocery store. These are easy to make, easy to freeze, and easy to reheat.

YIELD: 16 WAFFLES

4 tablespoons water

2 cups soy or rice milk

6 tablespoons vegetable oil

3 cups unbleached all-purpose flour

6 teaspoons baking powder

4 teaspoons granulated sugar

1 teaspoon salt

Preheat oven to 200°F, and heat a waffle iron according to the manufacturer's instructions.

In a large bowl, mix together the water, soy milk, and vegetable oil with a wire whisk until combined. In a medium bowl, combine the dry ingredients and add them to the water mixture. Stir until just combined. Do not overmix; a few lumps are fine.

Spray the inside of the waffle iron with dairy-free cooking spray. Pour on enough batter to spread to the edges. Close and bake according to manufacturer's instructions. Transfer the waffles to the warmed oven, and repeat with the remaining batter.

Tip: Freeze extra waffles by placing them in resealable plastic bags, with parchment or wax paper between each layer. Label with name and date, and freeze for up to 2 months. To reheat, unwrap waffles and toast on the low setting in a toaster.

Blueberry Waffles

Prepare Waffles recipe as directed. Pour 1 tablespoon fresh blueberries over the top of the batter after pouring it on the hot iron.

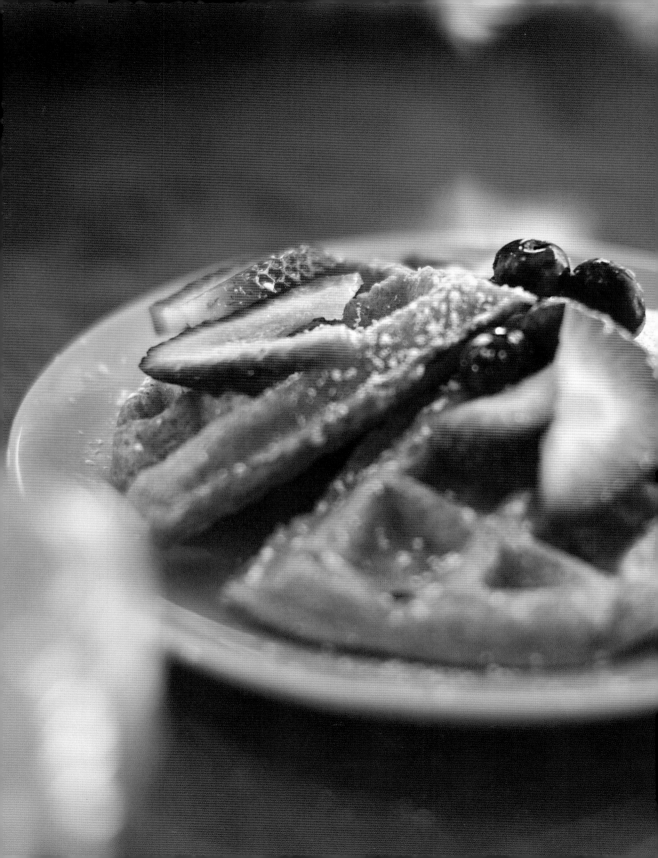

Whole-Wheat Waffles

These waffles are packed with flavor, and they freeze beautifully.

YIELD: 16 WAFFLES

2 tablespoons water

1¾ cups soy or rice milk

½ cup vegetable oil

2 cups whole-wheat flour

4 teaspoons baking powder

1 tablespoon light brown sugar

¼ teaspoon salt

Preheat oven to 200°F, and heat a waffle iron according to the manufacturer's instructions.

In a large bowl, mix together the water, soy milk, and vegetable oil with a wire whisk until combined. In a medium bowl, combine the flour, baking powder, brown sugar, and salt with a wire whisk, and add to the water mixture. Stir until just combined. Do not overmix; a few lumps are fine.

Spray the inside of the waffle iron with dairy-free cooking spray. Pour enough batter to spread to the edges. Close and bake according to manufacturer's instructions. Transfer the waffles to the warmed oven, and repeat with the remaining batter.

Tip: Freeze extra waffles by placing them in resealable plastic bags, with parchment or wax paper between each layer. Label with name and date, and freeze for up to 2 months. To reheat, unwrap waffles and toast on the low setting in a toaster.

Pancakes

I make a big batch of these pancakes and freeze the extras for busy mornings. People with food allergies can't order pancakes at a breakfast place, but they'll get the same taste with these.

YIELD: ABOUT 20 PANCAKES

2 cups all-purpose flour

4 tablespoons granulated sugar

4 teaspoons baking powder

¾ teaspoon salt

2 tablespoons water

4 tablespoons vegetable oil

2 cups soy or rice milk

Dairy-free cooking spray

Preheat a cast-iron griddle on medium heat until hot, and preheat oven to 200°F.

While the griddle is heating, combine the flour, sugar, baking powder, and salt with a wire whisk. In a large liquid measuring cup, combine the water, oil, and milk. Pour the water mixture into the dry ingredients, and mix with a wire whisk until just combined. Do not overmix; a few lumps are fine.

Spray the griddle liberally with dairy-free cooking spray (repeat this process each time you put down a new pool of batter). Pour about ¼ cup of batter onto the heated griddle, and cook until small bubbles start to form on top. Flip and cook the other side until light brown. Transfer the pancakes to the warmed oven, and repeat.

Note: I always spray the griddle first before pouring more batter on to prevent sticking. For evenly measured pancakes, use a cookie scooper.

Chocolate–Chip Pancakes

Prepare Pancakes recipe as directed. After pouring each ¼ cup of batter on the hot griddle, sprinkle 1 tablespoon dairy-free chocolate chips over the top of the batter.

Blueberry Pancakes

Prepare Pancakes recipe as directed. After pouring each ¼ cup of batter on the hot griddle, add a sprinkling of fresh or frozen blueberries over the top of the batter.

Tip: Freeze extras by placing pancakes in a resealable freezer bag, placing a sheet of parchment or wax paper between each layer. Label with name and date, and freeze for up to 2 months.

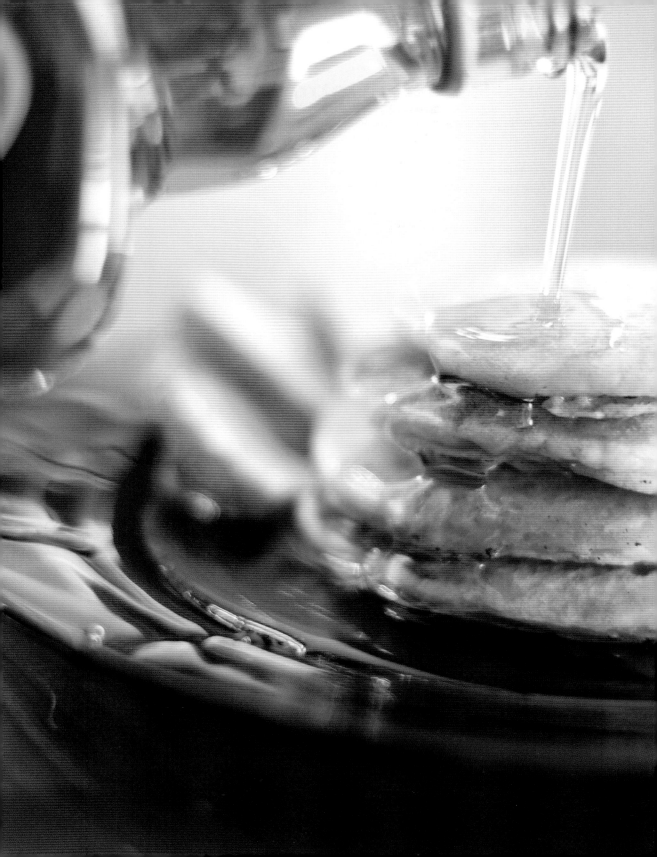

Heart-Healthy Oatmeal Pancakes

These pancakes are hearty, rich, and good for you, too. Freeze the extras for another morning.

YIELD: ABOUT 20 PANCAKES

1 cup quick-cooking oatmeal

1 cup whole-wheat flour

2 tablespoons granulated sugar

6 teaspoons baking powder

½ teaspoon salt

4 tablespoons water

1½ cups soy or rice milk

4 tablespoons vegetable oil

Preheat a cast-iron griddle pan on medium heat until hot, and preheat oven to 200°F.

Meanwhile, in a large bowl, combine the oatmeal, flour, sugar, baking powder, and salt with a wire whisk. In a large liquid measuring cup, combine the water, soy milk, and oil. Pour the water mixture into the dry ingredients, and mix with a wire whisk until just combined. Do not overmix; a few lumps are fine.

Spray the griddle liberally with dairy-free cooking spray (repeat this process each time you put down a new pool of batter). Pour about ¼ cup of batter onto the heated griddle, and cook until small bubbles start to form on top. Flip and cook the other side until light brown. Transfer the pancakes to warmed oven, and repeat.

Tip: Freeze extras by placing pancakes in a resealable freezer bag, placing a sheet of parchment or wax paper between each layer. Label with name and date, and freeze for up to 2 months.

Oatmeal Muffins

Soaking the raisins in soy milk plumps them up, making a more delicious muffin.

YIELD: 12 MUFFINS

1 cup raisins

¾ cup soy or rice milk

1 tablespoon water

½ cup vegetable oil

1 cup unbleached all-purpose flour

1 cup old-fashioned or quick-cooking oats

⅓ cup granulated sugar

3 teaspoons baking powder

½ teaspoon salt

½ teaspoon ground cinnamon

⅛ teaspoon ground nutmeg

Preheat oven to 400°F, and spray a 12-cup muffin pan with dairy-free baking spray. In a small bowl, stir together the raisins with the soy milk. Add the water and oil, and combine thoroughly. In a medium bowl, combine the flour, oats, sugar, baking powder, salt, cinnamon, and nutmeg with a wire whisk. Add the raisin–soy milk mixture to the dry ingredients, and stir until just moist. Do not overmix.

Divide the batter evenly among the prepared muffin cups, and bake for 18 to 20 minutes, or until lightly browned and an inserted cake tester comes out clean.

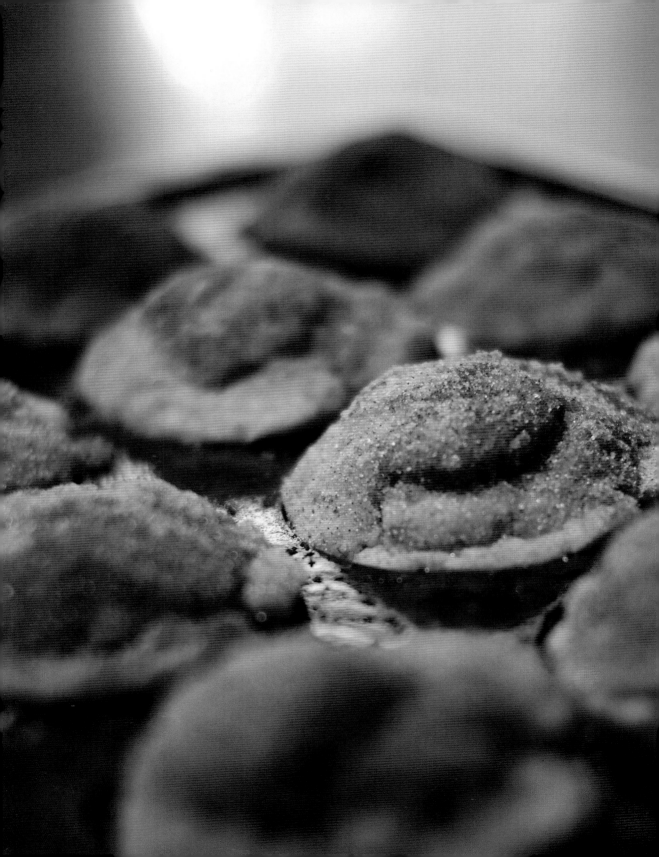

French Puff Muffins

These taste more like a yummy cinnamon doughnut than a muffin.

YIELD: 12 MUFFINS

Muffins

⅔ cup dairy-free margarine

1 tablespoon water

1 cup granulated sugar

3 cups unbleached all-purpose flour

1 teaspoon salt

½ teaspoon ground cinnamon

⅛ teaspoon ground nutmeg

3 teaspoons baking powder

1 cup soy or rice milk

Topping

½ cup melted dairy-free margarine

1 cup granulated sugar

2 teaspoons ground cinnamon

Preheat oven to 350°F, and spray a 12-cup muffin pan with dairy-free baking spray.

To make the muffins, in the bowl of a stand mixer fitted with the paddle attachment, combine the ⅔ cup margarine, water, and 1 cup sugar. In a medium bowl, combine the flour, salt, ½ teaspoon cinnamon, nutmeg, and baking powder with a wire whisk. Add the flour mixture and soy milk to the margarine–sugar mixture by thirds, alternating between each addition. Using a cookie scooper, place the batter into the prepared muffin pans. Bake for 15 to 20 minutes, or until an inserted cake tester comes out clean.

To make the topping, combine the 1 cup sugar and 2 teaspoons cinnamon in a small bowl, and place the melted ½ cup margarine in a small bowl. Remove the muffins from the pan and dip each in margarine, and then roll each muffin top in the cinnamon–sugar mixture.

Tip: These muffins are best when eaten the day they're made.

Berry Muffins

I like to try different berries in this recipe depending on what's in season or what we're in the mood for. Frozen berries work great too, and there's no need to defrost them.

YIELD: 12 MUFFINS

2 cups unbleached all-purpose flour

⅔ cup granulated sugar

2 teaspoons baking powder

¼ teaspoon salt

⅔ cup soy or rice milk

¼ cup vegetable oil or melted dairy-free margarine

½ teaspoon grated lemon zest

1 tablespoon fresh lemon juice

1 tablespoon water

½ teaspoon vanilla extract

1 cup fresh or frozen berries (e.g., blueberries, raspberries)

Granulated sugar, for sprinkling

Preheat oven to 400°F, and spray a 12-cup muffin pan with dairy-free baking spray.

In a medium bowl, combine the flour, sugar, baking powder, and salt with a wire whisk. In another medium bowl, combine the soy milk, vegetable oil or melted margarine, lemon zest, lemon juice, water, and vanilla with a spatula. Add the flour mixture to the soy milk mixture, and stir with a rubber spatula just until combined.

Lightly fold in the berries with a rubber spatula. Divide the batter evenly among 12 prepared muffin cups. Sprinkle the tops with granulated sugar, and bake for 20 minutes, or until an inserted cake tester comes out clean.

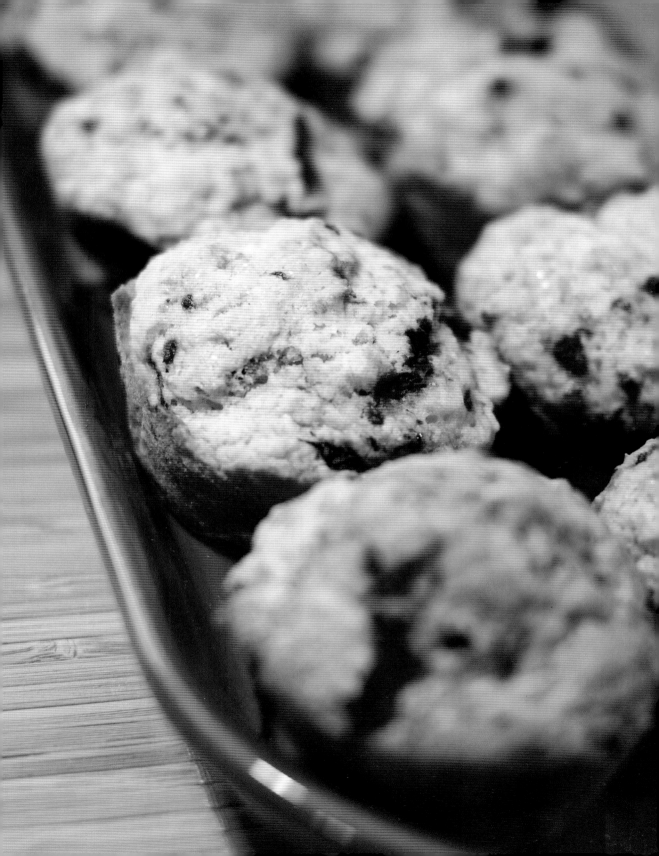

Corn Muffins

These little muffins are wonderful with chili. I also make them for my children's Thanksgiving parties at school.

YIELD: 12 MUFFINS

¼ cup dairy-free shortening (see page 15), melted

1½ cups dairy-free buttermilk (1½ cups soy or rice milk mixed with 1½ tablespoons white vinegar; let it sit for 5–10 minutes)

2 tablespoons water

1½ cups yellow cornmeal

½ cup unbleached all-purpose flour

2 teaspoons baking powder

1 teaspoon granulated sugar

½ teaspoon baking soda

½ teaspoon salt

Preheat oven to 450°F, and spray a 12-cup muffin pan with dairy-free baking spray.

In the bowl of a stand mixer fitted with the paddle attachment, thoroughly combine all ingredients. Fill the prepared muffin cups with batter, and bake for 18 to 20 minutes, or until an inserted cake tester comes out clean.

Breakfast Bran Muffins

I like the fact that these bran muffins are very straightforward. There's not a lot of chopped stuff, but just good, wholesome bran flavor. Of course, a little cinnamon and a few raisins don't hurt either.

YIELD: 12 MUFFINS

¾ cup soy or rice milk

1½ cups bran cereal (I use Kellogg's All-Bran; always check ingredient lists carefully)

1 tablespoon water

½ cup vegetable oil

¼ cup molasses

1¼ cups unbleached all-purpose flour

3 teaspoons baking powder

1 teaspoon ground cinnamon

½ teaspoon salt

½ cup raisins

Preheat oven to 400°F, and spray a 12-cup muffin pan with dairy-free baking spray. In a small bowl, pour the soy milk over the bran cereal, and let stand 2 minutes. Add the water, vegetable oil, and molasses to the bran mixture, and mix well.

In a separate medium bowl, combine the flour, baking powder, cinnamon, and salt with a wire whisk. Add the bran mixture to the dry ingredients, and stir until just combined; do not overmix. Stir in the raisins.

Divide the batter evenly among the prepared muffin cups, and bake for 18 to 20 minutes, or until lightly browned and an inserted cake tester comes out clean.

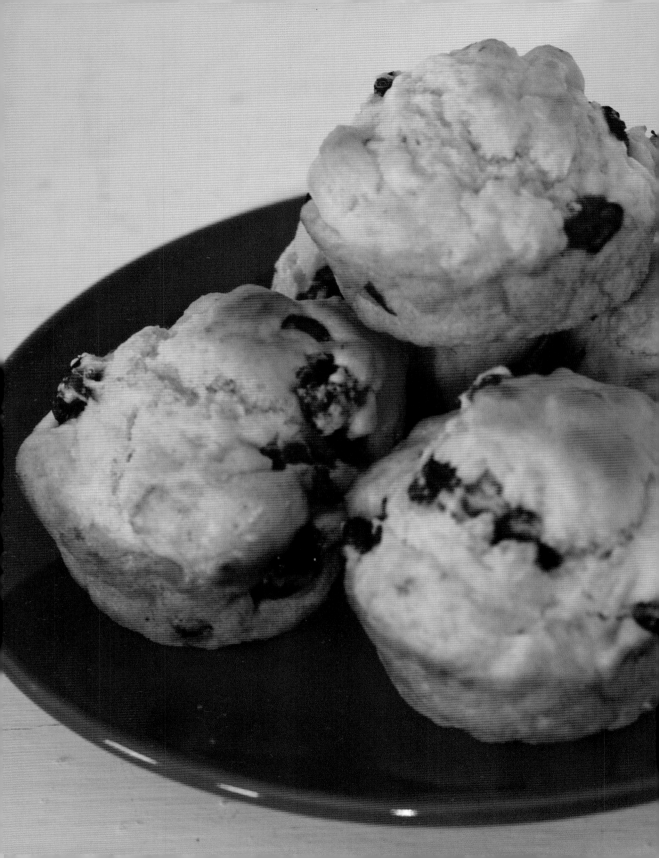

Cranberry–Orange Muffins

These are another holiday favorite at food gatherings. You could substitute defrosted frozen cranberries if fresh aren't available. Quickly defrost the cranberries by running them under hot water, and drain well.

YIELD: 12 MUFFINS

⅓ **cup vegetable oil**

¾ **cup soy or rice milk**

1 **tablespoon water**

1¾ **cups unbleached all-purpose flour**

½ **cup granulated sugar, divided**

2½ **teaspoons baking powder**

¾ **teaspoon salt**

1 **cup fresh cranberries, roughly chopped**

2 **teaspoons grated orange zest**

Preheat oven to 400°F, and generously spray a 12-cup muffin pan with dairy-free baking spray. In a large bowl, mix together the vegetable oil, soy milk, and water with a wire whisk. In a separate medium bowl, combine the flour, ¼ cup granulated sugar, baking powder, and salt with a wire whisk. Add the flour mixture to the vegetable oil mixture, and stir with a rubber spatula until just combined; do not overmix.

Set aside. In a small bowl, combine the cranberries, the remaining ¼ cup sugar, and the orange zest, and fold the mixture into the batter. Pour the batter into the prepared muffin cups, filling each cup ⅔ of the way full. Bake for 15 to 20 minutes, or until lightly browned and an inserted cake tester comes out clean.

Banana–Chocolate Chip Muffins

Kids love the combination of banana and chocolate. These are a huge hit with my family.

YIELD: 12 MUFFINS

2 medium bananas, mashed

2 tablespoons water

½ cup dairy-free margarine, melted

¼ cup dairy-free buttermilk (¼ cup soy or rice milk mixed with 1 teaspoon white vinegar; let it sit for 5–10 minutes)

2 cups unbleached all-purpose flour

⅔ cup granulated sugar

1½ teaspoons baking powder

1 teaspoon baking soda

¼ teaspoon salt

½ cup dairy-free mini chocolate chips

Preheat oven to 375°F, and spray a 12-cup muffin pan with dairy-free baking spray.

In the bowl of a stand mixer fitted with the paddle attachment, combine the mashed banana, water, melted margarine, and buttermilk until well incorporated.

In a medium bowl, combine the flour, sugar, baking powder, and baking soda with a wire whisk. Add the dry ingredients to the banana mixture, and mix well. Stir in the mini chocolate chips, and divide the batter evenly among the prepared muffin cups.

Bake for 15 to 20 minutes, or until golden brown and an inserted cake tester comes out clean.

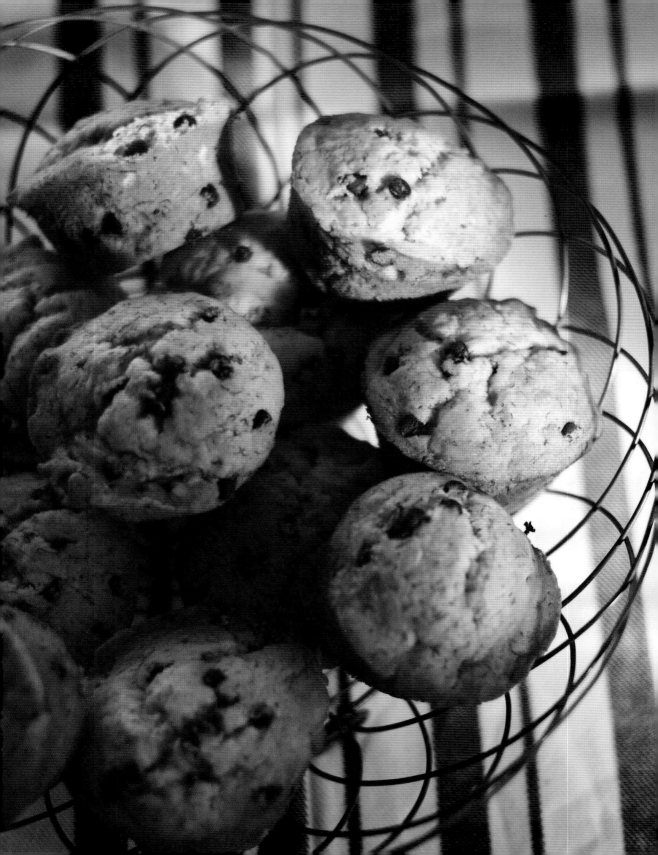

Apple Muffins

I like the texture of the chopped apples on the muffin top. Freeze the rest for later in the week or after school.

YIELD: 12 MUFFINS

Muffins

4 tablespoons dairy-free margarine, melted

¼ cup unsweetened applesauce

1 cup soy or rice milk

2 cups unbleached all-purpose flour

3 teaspoons baking powder

½ teaspoon salt

1 teaspoon ground cinnamon

¼ teaspoon ground nutmeg

½ cup granulated sugar

1½ cups diced, peeled apples, divided

Topping

¼ cup granulated sugar

½ teaspoon ground cinnamon

Preheat oven to 375°F, and spray a 12-cup muffin pan with dairy-free baking spray.

In the bowl of a stand mixer fitted with the paddle attachment, combine the melted margarine, applesauce, and soy milk. In a separate medium bowl, mix together the flour, baking powder, salt, the 1 teaspoon cinnamon, nutmeg, and the ½ cup sugar with a wire whisk. Add the dry ingredients to the apple mixture, and stir by hand with a rubber spatula until just until combined. Fold in the 1 cup chopped apple. Do not overmix.

Using a cookie scooper, fill the prepared muffin cups with batter, and top each with the remaining ½ cup diced apples.

To make the topping, in a small bowl, combine the ¼ cup sugar and the ½ teaspoon cinnamon, and sprinkle the mixture over the muffins. Bake for 20 to 25 minutes, or until an inserted cake tester comes out clean.

Tip: Freeze extra muffins for later by placing them in a resealable freezer bag. Label with name and date, and freeze for up to 2 months.

Blueberry Bran Muffins

For this recipe, I use Kellogg's All-Bran cereal. Make sure you always double-check food labels for changes in ingredients.

YIELD: 12 MUFFINS

3 cups bran flakes cereal

1¼ cups soy or rice milk

1 tablespoon water

5 tablespoons dairy-free margarine, melted

1¾ cups unbleached all-purpose flour

½ cup granulated sugar

¼ teaspoon salt

3 teaspoons baking powder

1 cup blueberries, fresh or frozen

Granulated sugar, for sprinkling

Preheat oven to 375°F, and spray a 12-cup muffin pan with dairy-free baking spray.

In a medium bowl, combine the cereal, soy milk, water, and margarine. Let stand for about 5 minutes. In another bowl, combine the flour, the ½ cup sugar, salt, and baking powder with a wire whisk. Add the wet cereal mixture to the flour mixture, and stir until just combined. Fold in the blueberries, and divide the batter evenly among the prepared muffin cups. Sprinkle with the remaining granulated sugar, and bake for 18 to 20 minutes, or until an inserted cake tester comes out clean.

Apple House Cinnamon Doughnuts

The Apple Haus, in Long Grove, Illinois, serves delicious apple cider doughnuts and apple pies. We stopped going there long ago because of John's allergies, but I never forgot how much I loved those doughnuts. I was determined to develop a recipe that closely matched those sweet and sugary treats. This recipe is the result of that mission, and it is fabulous. My son was so excited—not only could he have a doughnut for the first time in his life, but his were just as good as those at the Apple Haus.

YIELD: 12 DOUGHNUTS AND 12 HOLES

Doughnuts

Vegetable oil, for frying

¾ cup unsweetened applesauce

2 teaspoons vanilla extract

¾ cup granulated sugar

3 tablespoons dairy-free margarine, melted

4½–4¾ cups unbleached all-purpose flour

3½ teaspoons baking powder

1 teaspoon ground cinnamon

½ teaspoon ground nutmeg

½ teaspoon salt

1 cup soy or rice milk

Cinnamon sugar, for rolling

½ cup granulated sugar

2 teaspoons ground cinnamon

In a large, heavy pot, heat 2 to 3 inches of vegetable oil until a candy thermometer inserted in the oil reaches 375°F.

Meanwhile, in the bowl of a stand mixer fitted with the paddle attachment, combine the applesauce, vanilla, and ¾ cup sugar. Add the margarine, and mix well. In a separate medium bowl, combine the 4½ cups flour, baking powder, 1 teaspoon cinnamon, nutmeg, and salt with a wire whisk. Add the flour mixture and the soy milk alternately to the applesauce–margarine mixture. Add more flour, if needed, to make a smooth and not-too-sticky dough.

Transfer the dough to a lightly floured board. Knead for about 1 minute, and roll out to a ½-inch-thick circle. Dip a doughnut cutter into flour, and cut into the dough. Remove the trimmings and reroll, repeating the process.

Slide a few doughnuts into the hot oil, being careful not to crowd the pot. Fry until the doughnuts rise to the surface, about 2 minutes, and turn over with metal tongs to fry the other side. Doughnuts should be golden brown on both sides. Lift out the doughnuts with metal tongs and drain on paper towels.

Mix together the ½ cup sugar and the 2 teaspoons cinnamon. Place the cinnamon–sugar mixture in a brown paper lunch bag. Place the warm doughnuts, one at a time, in the brown bag, and shake to coat. Shake off excess sugar, and place on a serving platter. Repeat with remaining doughnuts.

Note: If you don't have a doughnut cutter, use a 3-inch biscuit cutter instead. To make the doughnut holes, use an empty, sterilized round medicine bottle without the cap. Poke the hole in the middle of the circle, and down the hole will pop. This is a time-tested trick I learned from my mom.

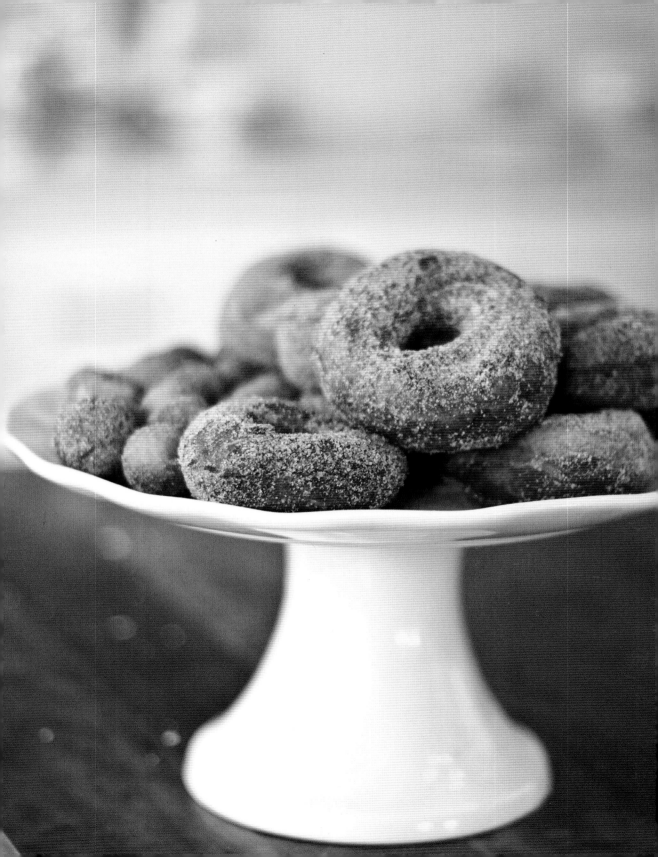

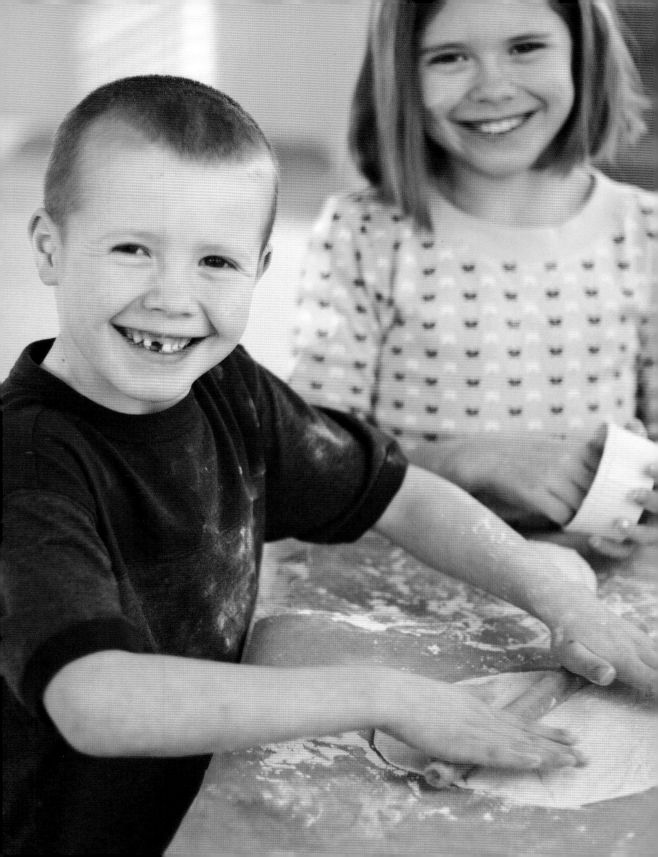

Biscuits, Scones, and Yeast Breads

Nothing improves a home-cooked meal quite like a loaf of freshly baked bread. People are usually intimidated by the idea of making yeast breads from scratch, but in reality, they are incredibly easy to make. Once you mix the yeast mixture with the dry ingredients, the breads practically make themselves. The only thing you really need is time to allow these breads to rise; the bake times are relatively short.

You'll find that you need little more than a spatula and bowl to mix together my biscuit and scone recipes, and they bake in minutes.

When I make more involved recipes, like Bakery-Style Bagels and Holiday Bread, my children love to help out. Kneading and handling the dough reminds them of playing with modeling clay, and it's a great tactile activity for them, too. It's so much fun to get your children to measure and mix ingredients, and even to get their hands a little dirty. You just might find kneading dough to be a therapeutic activity as well.

Currant Scones

Little currants are speckled throughout these scones. These are perfect with a cup of hot green tea.

YIELD: 12 SMALL SCONES

2 cups unbleached all-purpose flour

2 tablespoons granulated sugar

1 tablespoon baking powder

½ teaspoon salt

6 tablespoons dairy-free margarine, cut into small pieces

¾–1 cup soy or rice milk

⅓ cup currants

Preheat oven to 425°F, and line a baking sheet with parchment paper. Set aside. In a large bowl, combine the flour, sugar, baking powder, and salt using a wire whisk. Using a pastry blender or two knives, cut in the margarine until the mixture is crumbly. Make a well in the center of the flour mixture, and pour ¾ cup soy milk into the well, stirring with a rubber spatula until the dough just comes together. Add more soy milk, if needed. Stir in the currants.

Transfer the dough to a lightly floured surface. Knead about 15 times on the lightly floured surface. Using a pastry cutter, divide the dough in half, and shape each half into a flattened ball. Roll each ball out into a ½-inch-thick disk. Cut each circle into 6 wedges, and place each wedge on a prepared baking sheet. Bake for 18 to 20 minutes, until golden brown.

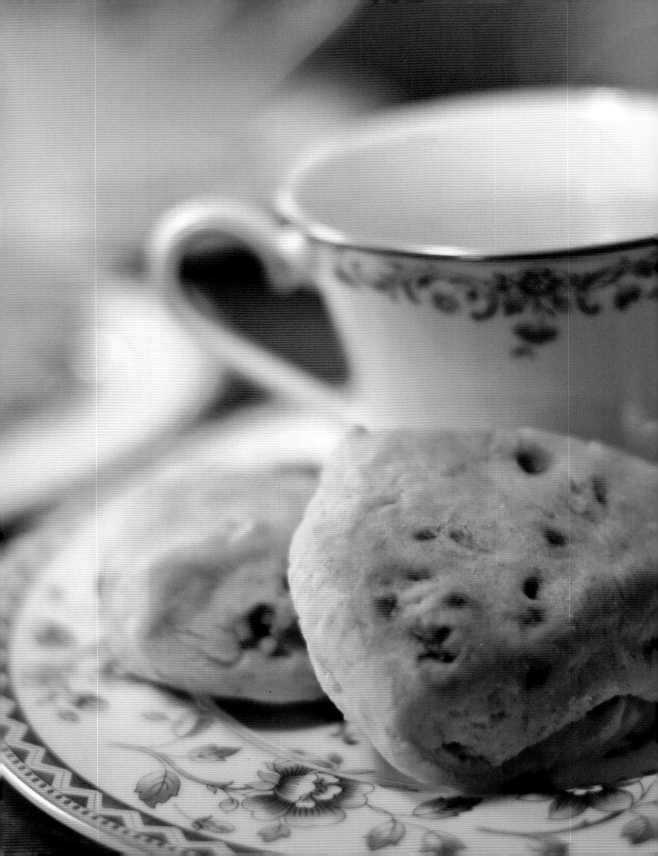

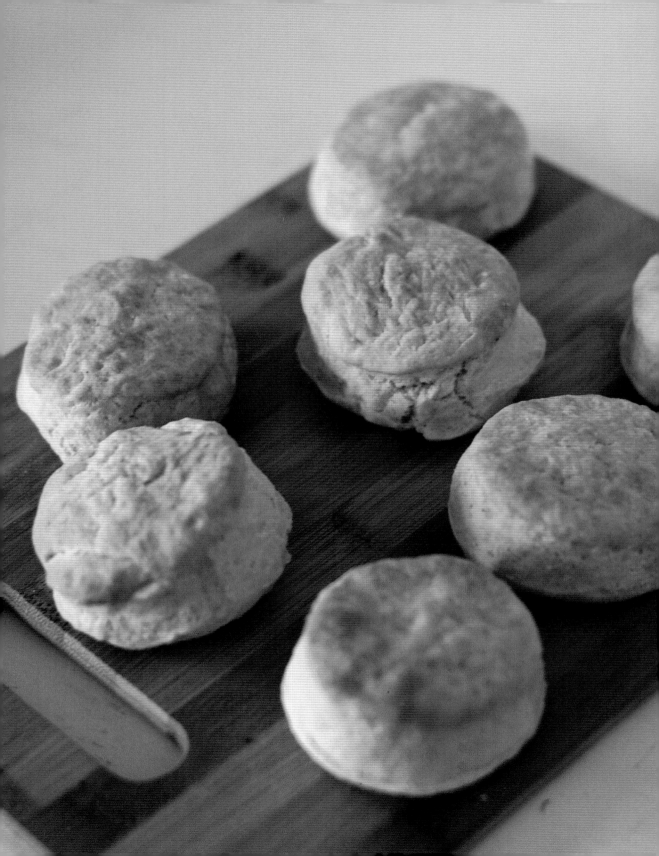

Dinner Biscuits

I really like biscuits with dinner, and freshly made biscuits are always better than the store-bought ones. Add the soy milk a little at a time until the dough is just starting to come together.

YIELD: 8 BISCUITS

2 cups unbleached all-purpose flour

1 tablespoon baking powder

1 teaspoon granulated sugar

½ teaspoon salt

¾–1 cup soy or rice milk

2 tablespoons dairy-free margarine, melted

Preheat oven to 425°F, and line a baking sheet with parchment paper. Set aside. In a medium bowl, combine the flour, baking powder, sugar, and salt with a wire whisk. Add the soy milk slowly, stirring with a rubber spatula until the dough just comes together and isn't too sticky. Turn onto a lightly floured surface, and knead 12 to 15 times, until the dough is soft and smooth.

Pat the dough into a circle about ½ inch thick. Using a 2-inch biscuit cutter, make 8 rounds, rerolling as necessary.

Brush the surface of each biscuit with melted dairy-free margarine, and bake for 15 to 20 minutes, or until lightly browned.

Cranberry– Orange Scones

I love freshly baked scones, and these are perfect, with just the right balance of sweet and tart. Scones are best when eaten right away.

YIELD: 12 SMALL SCONES

2½ cups unbleached all-purpose flour

2 tablespoons granulated sugar

1 tablespoon baking powder

½ teaspoon salt

6 tablespoons dairy-free margarine, cut into small pieces

3 teaspoons freshly squeezed orange juice

2 teaspoons grated orange zest

¾–1 cup soy or rice milk

¾ cup dried cranberries

1 tablespoon soy or rice milk, for brushing

Sugar, for sprinkling

Preheat oven to 425°F, and line a baking sheet with parchment paper. Set aside. In a medium bowl, combine the flour, sugar, baking powder, and salt with a wire whisk. Using a pastry blender, cut the margarine into the flour mixture until it is crumbly. Add the fresh orange juice and orange zest to the soy milk, and mix the orange–soy milk mixture into the flour mixture. Fold in the cranberries using a rubber spatula. Stir the dough until it just comes together and the dough is soft and not too sticky. If needed, add 1 to 2 tablespoons of additional flour.

Transfer the dough to a lightly floured surface, and knead about 15 times. Cut the dough in half, and shape each half into a ¾-inch-thick circle. Cut the dough into 6 wedges and place each on a baking sheet. Brush each wedge lightly with the soy milk, and sprinkle with sugar.

Bake for 18 to 20 minutes, until lightly golden brown.

Bakery-Style Bagels

When we go to a bagel shop, we pretty much know there are only a couple of allergen-free bagels John can have (plain and cinnamon–raisin). I thought, "Why not make them at home?" The dough is as easy to work with as kids' play dough, and kids of all ages will have fun shaping them into circles and poking holes through the center.

YIELD: 12 BAGELS

4½ cups unbleached all-purpose flour

2 packages active dry yeast

1½ cups warm water (about 110°F)

3½ tablespoons sugar

1 tablespoon salt

FOR BOILING

Water

1 tablespoon sugar

Preheat oven to 375°F, and line 2 baking sheets with parchment paper. In the bowl of a stand mixer fitted with the paddle attachment, combine 1½ cups of the flour and the yeast. Combine the 1½ cups warm water, the 3½ tablespoons sugar, and the salt in a separate bowl. Add the water mixture to the flour mixture, and mix with the stand mixer on low, using the dough hook attachment, for about 1 minute, scraping down the sides of the bowl. Turn the setting to high, and mix for about 3 to 4 more minutes. Stir in the remaining flour until the dough comes together and is somewhat stiff.

Turn the dough onto a floured board, and knead until smooth and elastic, about 5 minutes. Cover with a kitchen towel, and let rest about 10 minutes.

Cut the dough into 12 portions, and shape each into a ball. Using your finger, punch a hole in the middle of each ball. Cover, and let rise another 10 to 15 minutes.

Fill a large, heavy pot with the water and 1 tablespoon sugar, and bring to a boil. Reduce heat to a simmer, drop in 4 bagels at a time, and cook for 5 to 7 minutes, turning once. Don't overcrowd the pot. Use metal tongs to remove the bagels from the pot, and drain them on paper towels. Place the drained bagels on prepared baking sheets, and bake for about 30 minutes, or until golden brown.

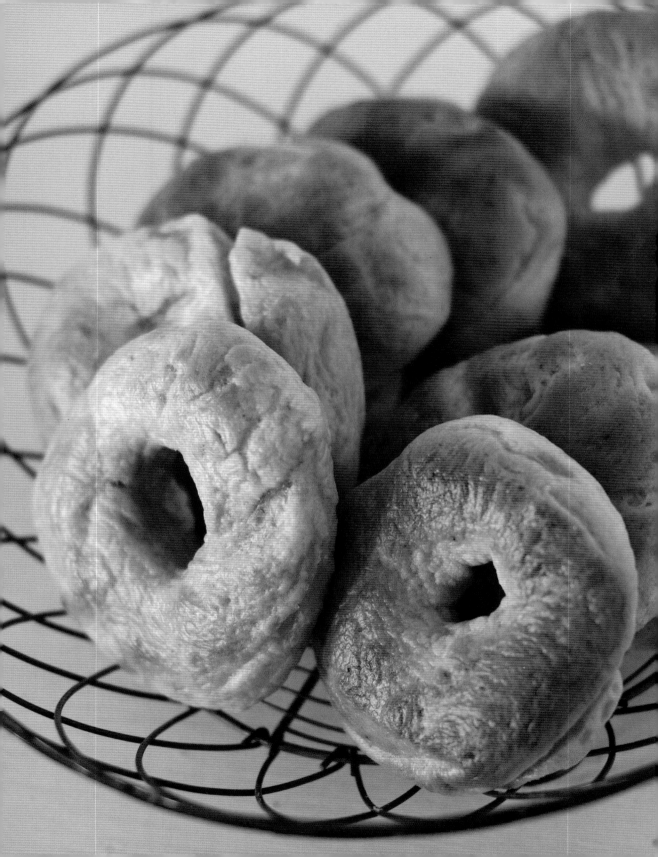

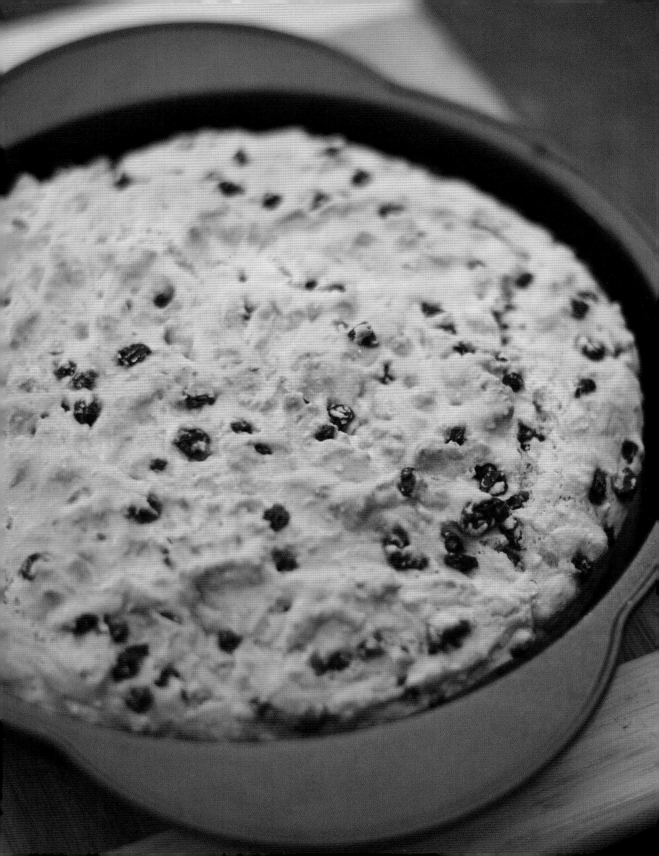

Irish Soda Bread

I love the simplicity of Irish Soda Bread. Make it with potato soup during the winter months, and with corned beef and potatoes for St. Patrick's Day. Add up to ¼ cup additional currants if you like a sweeter soda bread.

YIELD: 1 ROUND LOAF

3 cups unbleached all-purpose flour

2 tablespoons brown sugar

2 teaspoons baking powder

1 teaspoon baking soda

1 teaspoon salt

1½ cups dairy-free butter-milk (2 cups soy or rice milk mixed with 2 tablespoons white vinegar; let it sit for 5–10 minutes)

½ cup currants

¾ teaspoon caraway seeds

Preheat oven to 350°F, and spray a 9-inch cake pan with dairy-free baking spray. In a large bowl, combine the flour, brown sugar, baking powder, baking soda, and salt with a wire whisk. Slowly add the buttermilk, and stir with a rubber spatula until just combined. Stir in the currants and caraway seeds.

Place the batter into the prepared pan, and bake for 30 to 40 minutes, or until lightly browned.

Old-Fashioned White Bread

The smell of freshly baked bread in the oven is comforting. Making your own bread is easier than you think, and worth the extra effort. Eat one loaf now, and freeze the other for later.

YIELD: 2 LOAVES

6–6¼ cups unbleached all-purpose flour, divided

1 package active dry yeast

2 cups soy or rice milk

2 tablespoons granulated sugar

2 tablespoons dairy-free shortening (see page 15)

1½ teaspoons salt

In the bowl of a stand mixer fitted with the dough hook attachment, combine 2½ cups of the flour and the yeast with a wire whisk. Set aside. In a medium saucepan, heat the soy milk, sugar, shortening, and salt until warm, about 110°F. Add the soy milk mixture to the flour mixture, and beat on low for about 1 minute. Scrape down the bowl's sides with a rubber spatula, and then beat on high for an additional minute.

Stir in the remaining flour, 1 cup at a time, to make a pliable dough. Turn the dough onto a floured board, and knead 10 minutes, until the dough is smooth and elastic. Transfer the dough ball to a bowl sprayed with dairy-free baking spray, turning the dough to coat all sides. Cover with a kitchen towel, and let rise until doubled in bulk, about 1 hour. Punch the dough down, and divide into 2 portions.

Shape each portion into a ball, and place each on a lightly floured board. Cover with a kitchen towel, and let rest about 5 minutes. Place the dough into two 8-inch loaf pans sprayed generously with dairy-free baking spray. Cover the pans with kitchen towels, and let rise until doubled in bulk, 30 to 45 minutes.

Preheat oven to 375°F. Bake for 40 to 50 minutes, or until the tops are browned and make a hollow sound when tapped. Cool completely on a wire rack.

Tip: Freeze bread by wrapping well in plastic wrap, and then aluminum foil. Label with name and date; freeze for up to 2 months.

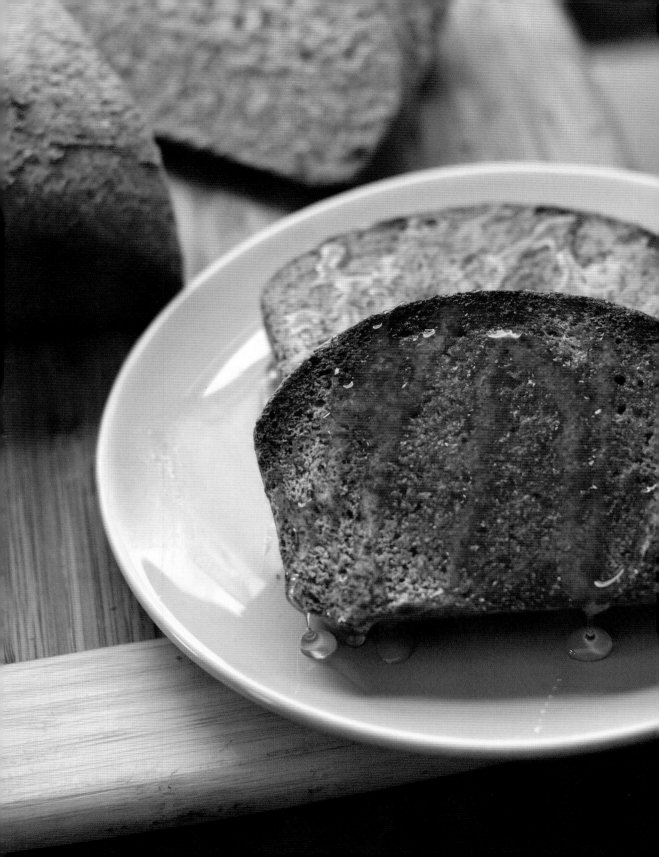

Old-Fashioned Whole-Wheat Bread

This is one of my favorite breads to make. It is delicious toasted and spread with dairy-free margarine and honey.

YIELD: 2 LOAVES

4–4½ cups whole-wheat flour, divided

2 packages active dry yeast

2 cups soy or rice milk

⅓ cup light brown sugar

2 tablespoons dairy-free shortening (see page 15)

1½ teaspoons salt

In the bowl of a stand mixer fitted with the dough hook attachment, combine 2½ cups of the flour and the yeast with a wire whisk. In a medium saucepan, heat the soy milk, sugar, shortening, and salt until warm, about 110°F. Add the soy milk mixture to the flour mixture, and beat on low for about 1 minute. Scrape down the bowl's sides with a rubber spatula. Beat on high for an additional minute.

Stir in the remaining flour, 1 cup at a time, to make a stiff, but pliable, dough. Turn the dough onto a floured board, and knead 10 minutes, until the dough is smooth and elastic. Transfer the dough to a bowl sprayed with dairy-free baking spray, turning to coat all sides. Cover with a kitchen towel, and let rise until doubled in bulk, about 1 hour. Transfer the dough ball to a bowl sprayed with dairy-free baking spray, turning the dough to coat all sides. Cover with a kitchen towel, and let rise until doubled in bulk, about 1 hour. Punch the dough down, and divide into 2 portions.

Shape each portion into a ball, and place each on a lightly floured board. Cover with a kitchen towel, and let rest about 5 minutes. Place the dough into two 8-inch loaf pans sprayed generously with dairy-free baking spray. Cover the pans with kitchen towels, and let rise until doubled in bulk, 30 to 45 minutes.

Preheat oven to 375°F. Bake for 35 to 45 minutes. Cool slightly, and then remove from pans onto wire rack to cool completely.

Holiday Bread

This large loaf is braided like a challah loaf, but it tastes like a delicious Italian loaf bread. You could separate the dough into two large loaves, or follow the recipe below to make a braided loaf. Either way, it will be a gorgeous bread that is crusty on the outside, and soft and chewy on the inside.

YIELD: 12 SERVINGS

2 packages active dry yeast

½ cup warm water (about 110°F)

1 cup soy or rice milk

¼ cup dairy-free margarine

1 tablespoon granulated sugar

2 teaspoons salt

4¾–5 cups unbleached all-purpose flour

2 tablespoons room-temperature water

1 tablespoon soy or rice milk, for brushing

Combine the yeast and warm water with a wire whisk, and set aside. In a small saucepan, heat the soy milk, margarine, sugar, and salt until dissolved. Cool slightly. In the bowl of a stand mixer fitted with the dough hook attachment, combine the salt and 2 cups of the flour with the soy milk mixture, and beat well. Add the yeast mixture and 2 tablespoons water, and beat well. Stir in the remaining flour on low until the dough becomes soft and pliable.

Transfer the dough onto a floured surface, and knead about 10 minutes. Shape into a ball, and place in a bowl sprayed with dairy-free baking spray, turning once to coat the ball. Cover with a kitchen towel, and let rise until doubled in bulk, about 1 hour. Punch down the dough and divide it into 3 balls. Cover again with a kitchen towel, and let rest 10 minutes. Roll each third of the dough into 16-inch-long strands. Braid the strands together, and tuck in the ends. Place the loaf on a parchment-lined baking sheet. Cover, and let rise 30 minutes.

Preheat oven to 375°F. Brush the loaf with 1 tablespoon soy milk, and bake for 40 to 50 minutes, or until golden brown.

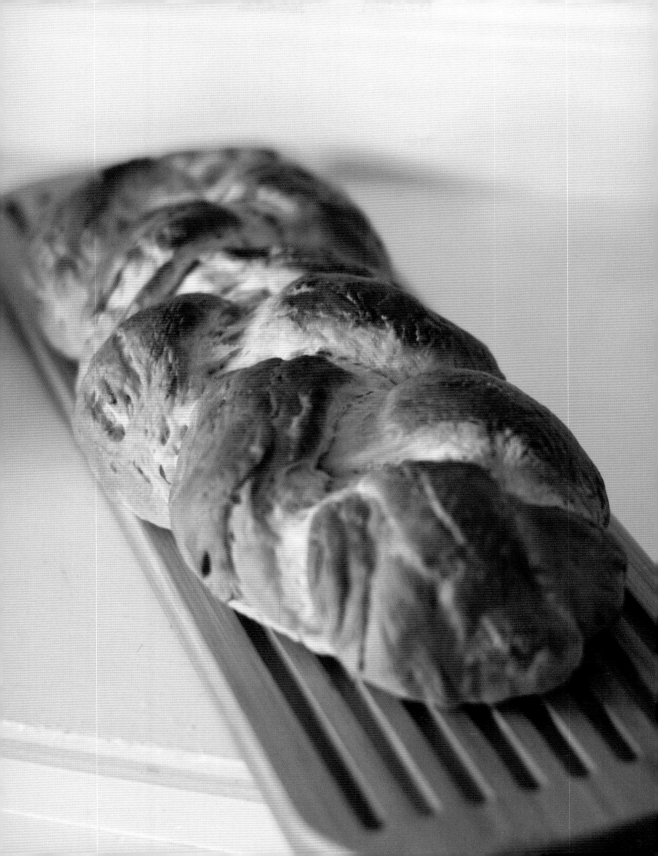

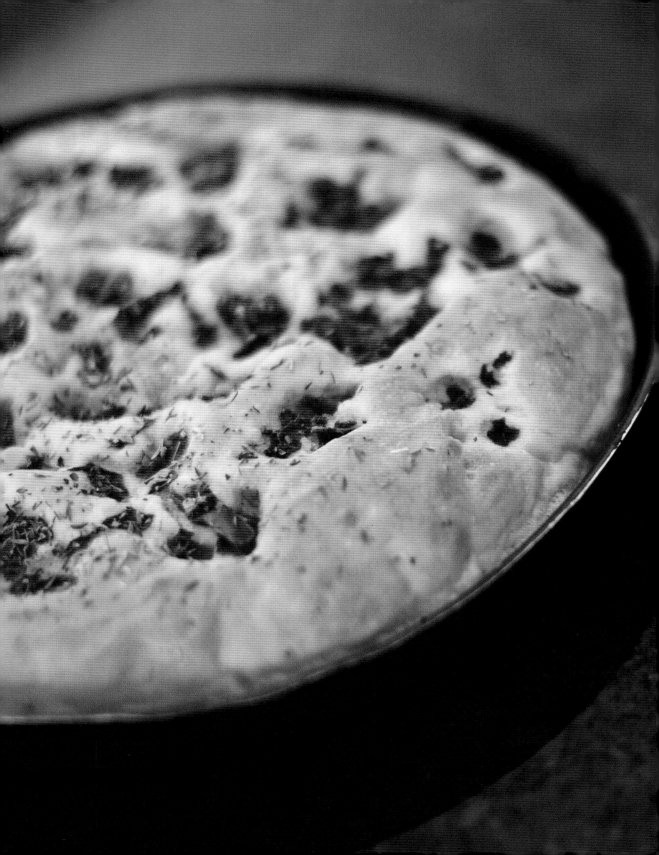

Italian Focaccia Bread

I've made this bread for years, and it never fails me. It is easy to make and can be varied with different herbs, fresh or dried. You could even throw in Kalamata olives, too.

YIELD: 6 SERVINGS

1⅓ cups warm water (about 110°F)

1 package active dry yeast

5 tablespoons olive oil, divided

3¼ cups unbleached all-purpose flour

1½ teaspoons salt

2 cups canned diced tomatoes, drained

1 tablespoon dried rosemary, crumbled

¼ teaspoon kosher salt, for sprinkling

Combine the warm water, yeast, and 3 tablespoons of the olive oil in a liquid measuring cup with a wire whisk. In a medium bowl, combine the flour and 1½ teaspoons salt with a wire whisk, and slowly mix this dry mixture into the water mixture with a rubber spatula. Stir until the mixture is well incorporated, and then mix quickly for about 2 minutes. Cover with plastic wrap, and let rise in a warm place until doubled in size, about 1 hour.

Using a brush, spread 1 tablespoon olive oil on the bottom and up the sides of a 14-inch round pizza pan. Transfer the dough into the pan, and press the dough into the pan and up the sides. Cover the dough with plastic wrap sprayed with dairy-free baking spray, and let rise again until doubled in size, 30 to 45 minutes.

Preheat oven to 425°F. Using your fingers, poke holes in the surface of the focaccia. Drizzle the remaining 1 tablespoon olive oil evenly over the top. Sprinkle with the tomatoes, rosemary, and kosher salt, and bake for 20 to 25 minutes, or until the top is golden brown. Cool on a wire rack for about 10 minutes, and cut into slices.

Quick Pizza Dough

Since you can't order in a pizza, make it at home! This dough is ridiculously easy to throw together, and you can freeze it, wrapped well and placed in a resealable plastic bag, for up to 2 months. Top with fresh tomato sauce, soy cheese, and fresh veggies. If you are going to use soy cheese, read the labels carefully, because a lot of imitation and soy cheeses contain milk products.

YIELD: ONE 14-INCH PIZZA OR SIX MINI PIZZAS

1 package active dry yeast

1 cup warm water (about 110°F)

1½ teaspoons granulated sugar

1 teaspoon salt

2 tablespoons olive oil

2½ cups unbleached all-purpose flour

Preheat oven to 425°F. Combine the yeast and warm water with a wire whisk, and set aside. In the bowl of a stand mixer fitted with the dough hook attachment, combine the sugar, salt, olive oil, and flour with the yeast mixture for about 1 minute, or until combined. Set aside to rest for 5 minutes.

Turn the dough onto a floured board, and knead about 15 times. Cut into desired portions.

Place the dough on a nonstick baking pan. Top as desired and bake for about 20 minutes, or until the crust is golden and the topping is warmed through.

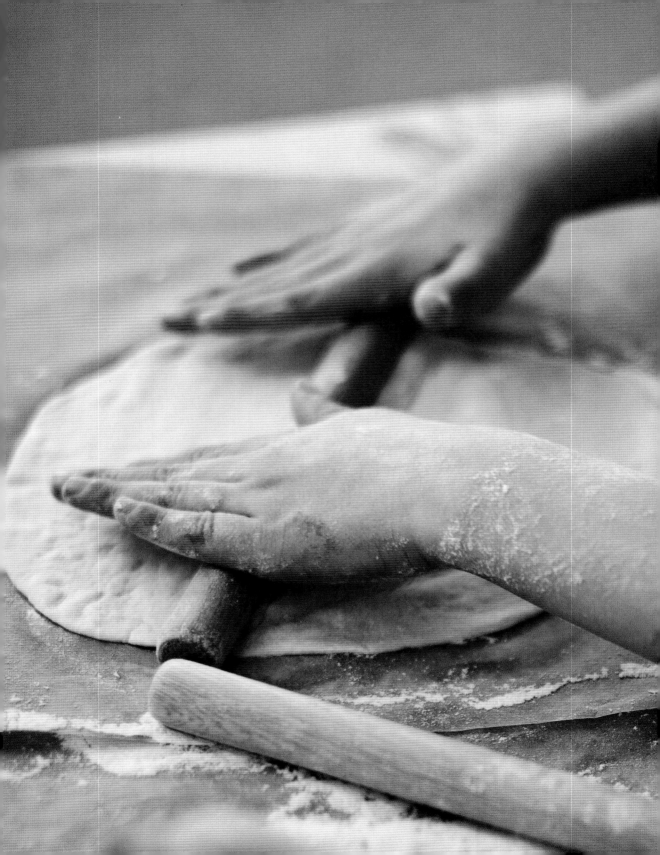

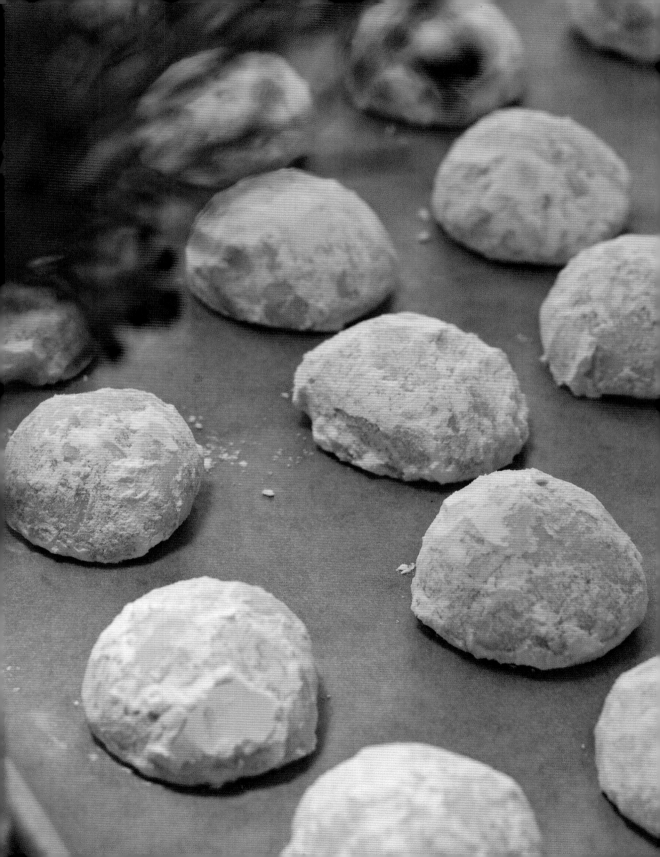

Cookies and Bars

Making cookies is a great way to create timeless childhood memories for your children. I have so many wonderful memories of making Christmas and chocolate chip cookies with my mom. I never wanted John to be robbed of the opportunity to pull up a chair to the kitchen counter and stir and sample fresh cookie batter. An added bonus of these recipes is all kids can eat the batter as much as they want, since the batter is egg free. Just like the rest of my kids, John can have a real taste of childhood.

I make a lot of these cookies and bars for class parties, bake sales, and after-school treats. They never fail to please and fill the kitchen and house with delicious and enticing aromas. The best part is the children in our neighborhood don't know the difference between these cookies and more traditional ones. They just know they taste wonderful.

Chocolate Chip Cookies

This is by far my most requested recipe. Everyone *loves these cookies—even those who don't have food allergies. Double the recipe to keep the cookie jar filled for treat days at school and after-school snacks.*

YIELD: 2 DOZEN COOKIES

⅔ cup dairy-free shortening (see page 15)

½ cup brown sugar

½ cup granulated sugar

¼ cup unsweetened applesauce

1 teaspoon best-quality vanilla extract

1¾ cups unbleached all-purpose flour

½ teaspoon baking soda

½ teaspoon salt

1 cup dairy-free mini chocolate chips

Preheat oven to 375°F, and line a baking sheet with parchment paper. In the bowl of a stand mixer fitted with the paddle attachment, combine the shortening, sugars, applesauce, and vanilla until smooth. In a medium bowl, combine the flour, baking soda, and salt with a wire whisk. Add the flour mixture to the shortening mixture, and stir until just combined. Stir in the chocolate chips.

Use a cookie scooper to place the batter onto the prepared baking sheet. Bake for 12 to 15 minutes, or until lightly browned. Cool completely on the baking sheet.

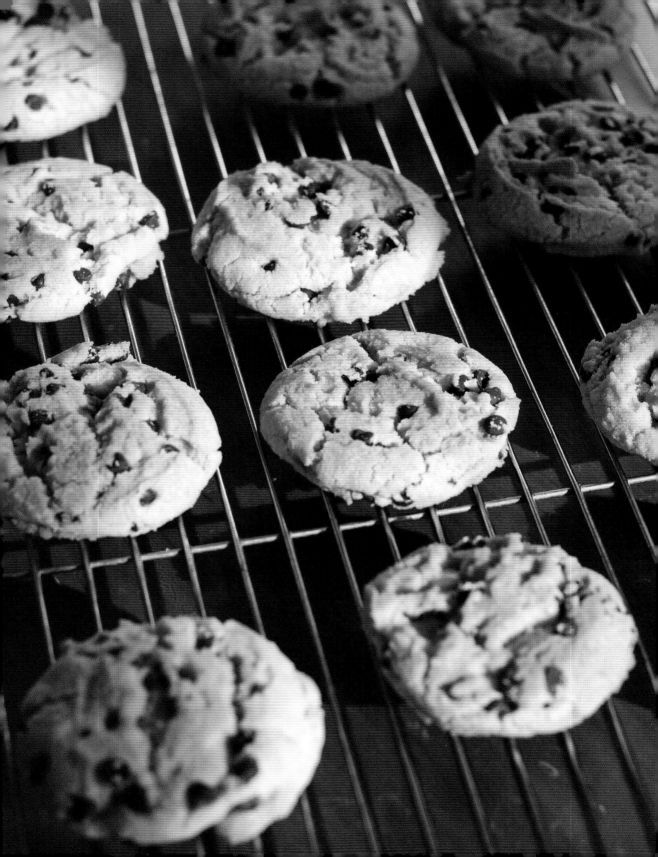

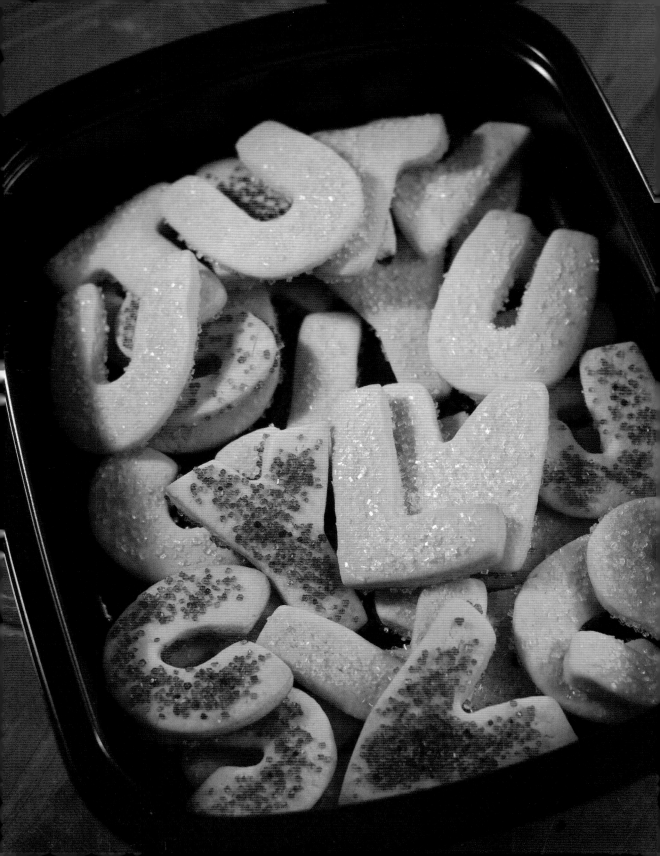

Cutout Sugar Cookies

I always make a big batch of these cookies for holidays and as treats for class parties. Precut and bake your desired shapes (think Halloween, Valentine's Day, etc.), and bring them to your child's class for a party activity. Set out bowls of colored icing and allergen-safe sprinkles to decorate. These cookies have a dual role: both classroom activity and treat!

YIELD: 2 DOZEN COOKIES, DEPENDING ON COOKIE CUTTER SIZE

¾ cup dairy-free shortening (see page 15)

1 cup granulated sugar

½ cup unsweetened applesauce

1½ teaspoons vanilla extract

2¾ cups unbleached all-purpose flour

1 teaspoon baking powder

½ teaspoon salt

1 recipe Classic Cookie Icing (recipe follows)

Preheat oven to 400°F, and line 2 baking sheets with parchment paper. Set aside. In the bowl of a stand mixer fitted with the paddle attachment, thoroughly combine the shortening, sugar, applesauce, and vanilla. In a separate medium bowl, combine the flour, baking powder, and salt with a wire whisk. Add the flour mixture to the shortening mixture, and mix on low until combined. Chill the dough in the refrigerator for 1 hour or more.

Roll the dough to a ¼-inch thickness on a floured board. Dip cookie cutters in some flour, cut out the desired shapes, and place the cut shapes on the baking sheets. Bake for 8 to 10 minutes, or until very light golden. Cool completely on the baking sheets.

Classic Cookie Icing

1 cup confectioners' sugar, sifted

¾ teaspoon vanilla extract

1–2 tablespoons soy or rice milk

Food coloring (optional)

Combine the confectioners' sugar and vanilla extract in a small bowl. Stir in just enough soy or rice milk to make a thin glaze.

Dairy-Free Sour Cream Cookies

Thank goodness for dairy-free sour cream! You can't even tell this cookie is dairy- and egg-free.

YIELD: 2 DOZEN COOKIES

½ cup dairy-free shortening (see page 15)

1 cup granulated sugar

¼ cup unsweetened applesauce

1 teaspoon vanilla extract

2¾ cups unbleached all-purpose flour

1 teaspoon baking powder

½ teaspoon baking soda

¼ teaspoon salt

¼ teaspoon nutmeg

½ cup dairy-free sour cream

Crystallized sugar, for sprinkling

In the bowl of a stand mixer fitted with the paddle attachment, combine the shortening, sugar, applesauce, and vanilla until thoroughly combined. In a separate medium bowl, combine the flour, baking powder, baking soda, salt, and nutmeg with a wire whisk. Add the flour mixture to the shortening mixture, and mix well. Add the sour cream, and mix on medium for 1 to 2 minutes, or until smooth.

Divide the dough, and transfer it to a lightly floured surface. Roll the dough to a ¼-inch thickness, and cut dough rounds using a 1-inch round cookie cutter.

Preheat oven to 425°F, and line a baking sheet with parchment paper. Using a spatula, transfer the dough rounds to the prepared baking sheet, and sprinkle each cookie with the crystallized sugar. Bake for 7 to 10 minutes, or until very lightly browned. Cool completely.

Chewy Double Chocolate Cookies

The taste of a Little Debbie snack cake in a dairy-, egg-, and nut-free cookie!

YIELD: 2 DOZEN COOKIES

⅔ cup dairy-free margarine

1 cup granulated sugar

¼ cup unsweetened applesauce

⅔ cup dairy-free buttermilk (1 cup soy or rice milk mixed with 1 tablespoon white vinegar; let it sit for 5–10 minutes)

1 teaspoon vanilla extract

2 cups unbleached all-purpose flour

½ cup cocoa powder

½ teaspoon baking soda

½ teaspoon salt

1 cup dairy-free mini chocolate chips

In the bowl of a stand mixer fitted with the paddle attachment, combine the margarine, sugar, applesauce, buttermilk, and vanilla. In a separate medium bowl, combine the flour, cocoa powder, baking soda, and salt with a wire whisk. Add the flour mixture to the margarine mixture, and mix on low for about 1 minute to combine. Increase the speed to medium high, and beat for 2 to 3 more minutes.

Preheat oven to 400°F, and line a baking sheet with parchment paper. Use a cookie scooper to place the dough onto the baking sheet. Bake for 7 to 10 minutes, or until set. Cool completely on the baking sheet.

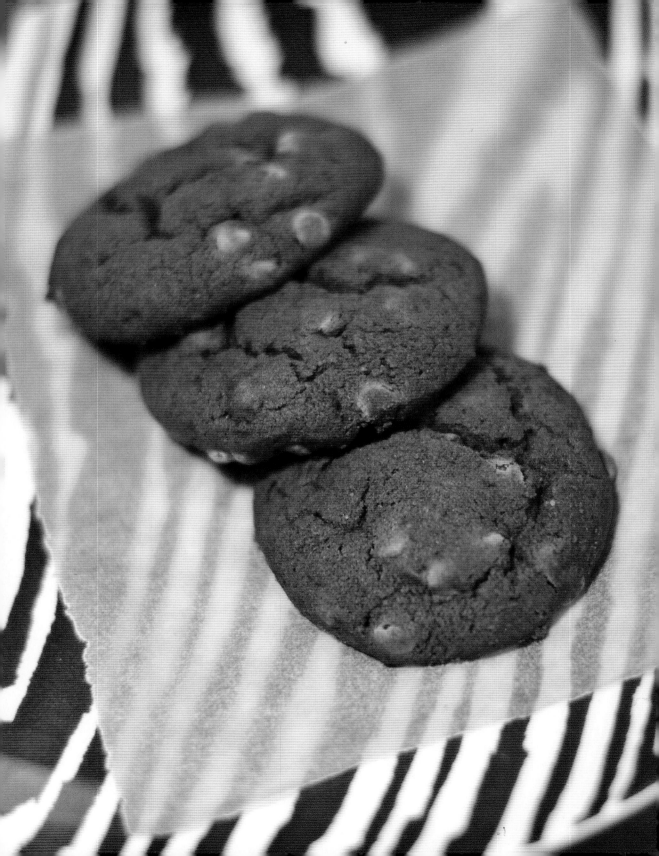

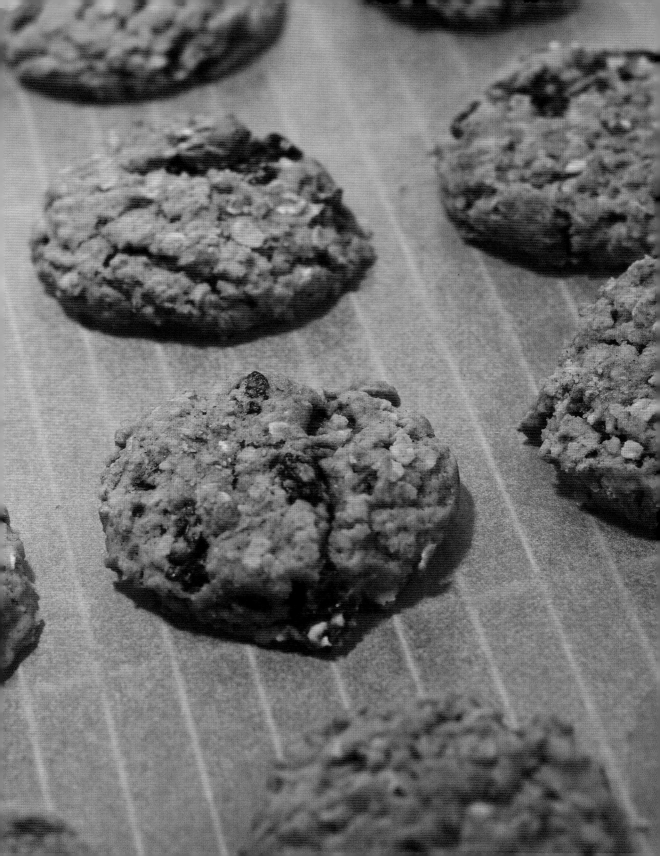

Oatmeal–Raisin Cookies

I make these as a special treat for my nephews, Devin and James. (Their mom, Chris, is a pretty big fan of these cookies, too.) If they make the trip to visit me in Chicago, I make sure to have these on hand. They are soft and chewy, and simply the best oatmeal cookie I've ever tasted.

YIELD: 2 DOZEN COOKIES

½ cup dairy-free shortening (see page 15)

1 cup granulated sugar

½ cup unsweetened applesauce

⅓ cup molasses

2 cups unbleached all-purpose flour

1 teaspoon ground cinnamon

1 teaspoon baking soda

½ teaspoon salt

2 cups quick-cooking or old-fashioned oats

1 cup raisins

Preheat oven to 400°F. In the bowl of a stand mixer fitted with the paddle attachment, combine the shortening, sugar, applesauce, and molasses until smooth. In a medium bowl, combine the flour, cinnamon, baking soda, and salt with a wire whisk. Add the flour mixture to the shortening mixture, and beat well.

Line a baking sheet with parchment paper. Stir the oats and raisins into the cookie dough with a rubber spatula. Use a cookie scooper to place the dough onto the prepared baking sheet. Bake for 7 to 10 minutes, or until lightly browned. Remove from the oven, press down slightly on the dough, and let cool completely on the baking sheet.

Oatmeal–Chocolate Chip Cookies

Prepare Oatmeal–Raisin Cookie recipe as directed, but substitute 1 cup dairy-free mini chocolate chips for the raisins.

Cranberry–Chocolate Drop Cookies

As a runner, I am drawn to granola and power bars. These remind me of my favorite nutrition bar, which is packed with little bits of dairy-free semisweet chocolate and fresh cranberries. If cranberries aren't in season, use frozen cranberries that have been quickly defrosted under warm running water.

YIELD: 2 DOZEN COOKIES

½ cup dairy-free margarine

1 cup granulated sugar

¾ cup packed brown sugar

¼ cup soy or rice milk

2 tablespoons orange juice

1 teaspoon grated orange zest

¼ cup unsweetened applesauce

3¼ cups unbleached all-purpose flour

1 teaspoon baking powder

½ teaspoon salt

¼ teaspoon baking soda

1 cup dairy-free chocolate chips

2½ cups coarsely chopped fresh cranberries

In the bowl of a stand mixer fitted with the paddle attachment, combine the margarine and sugars together until light and fluffy. Add the soy milk, orange juice, orange zest, and applesauce to the mixture, and mix thoroughly.

In a separate medium bowl, combine the flour, baking powder, salt, and baking soda using a wire whisk. Add the flour mixture to the margarine mixture, and blend well. Stir in the chocolate chips and chopped cranberries.

Preheat oven to 375°F, and line 2 baking sheets with parchment paper. Use a cookie scooper to place the dough onto the prepared baking sheets. Bake for 12 to 15 minutes, or until lightly browned. Cool completely on the baking sheets.

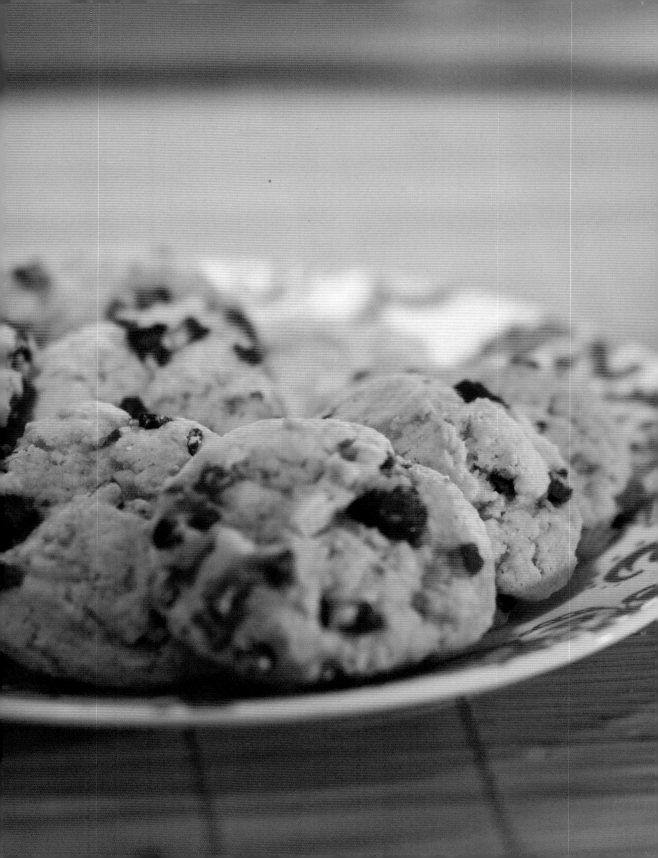

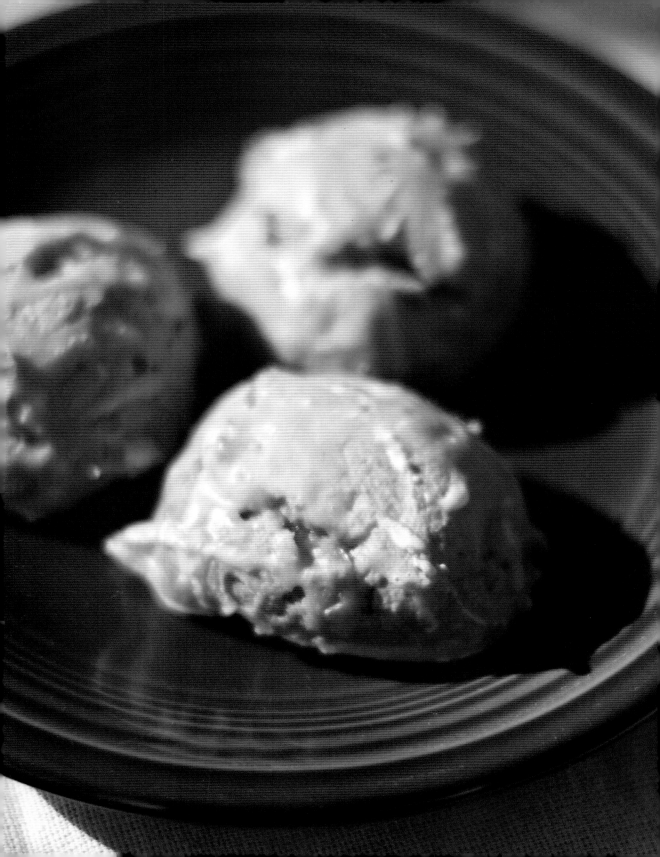

Pumpkin Cookies

These are little buttons of pumpkin with a creamy glaze spread on top. It's a perfect pumpkin treat.

YIELD: 2 DOZEN COOKIES

½ cup dairy-free shortening (see page 15)

1½ cups light brown sugar

½ cup unsweetened applesauce

1 (15-ounce) can pumpkin purée (not pumpkin pie filling)

3 cups unbleached all-purpose flour

1 tablespoon baking powder

1 teaspoon ground cinnamon

¼ teaspoon ground nutmeg

¼ teaspoon ground ginger

¼ teaspoon salt

Classic Icing (recipe follows)

In the bowl of a stand mixer fitted with the paddle attachment, thoroughly combine the shortening, sugar, applesauce, and pumpkin. In a separate medium bowl, combine the flour, baking powder, cinnamon, nutmeg, ginger, and salt with a wire whisk. Add the flour mixture to the shortening mixture, and stir until just combined.

Preheat oven to 400°F, and line 2 baking sheets with parchment paper. Use a cookie scooper to place batter onto the prepared baking sheets. Bake for 12 to 15 minutes, or until lightly browned. Remove from the oven, and cool on a wire rack. Frost the cookies with Classic Icing.

Classic Icing

2 cups confectioners' sugar

1 teaspoon good-quality vanilla extract

3–4 tablespoons soy or rice milk, as needed to thin icing

Blend all ingredients together in a small bowl with a wire whisk. Drizzle over Pumpkin Cookies, or dip each cookie into the bowl of icing.

Molasses Cookies

My brother-in-law, Jim, loves these cookies, and each Christmas, he asks me to send them to him in Kentucky. It is a delicious cookie with a classic molasses taste.

YIELD: 2 DOZEN

¾ cup dairy-free shortening (see page 15)

1 cup light brown sugar

¼ cup unsweetened applesauce

¼ cup molasses

2½ cups unbleached all-purpose flour

2 teaspoons baking soda

1 teaspoon ground cinnamon

1 teaspoon ground ginger

¼ teaspoon ground cloves

⅛ teaspoon salt

½ cup granulated sugar, for dipping

¼ cup water

In the bowl of a stand mixer fitted with the paddle attachment, thoroughly combine the shortening, brown sugar, applesauce, and molasses. In a separate medium bowl, combine the flour, baking soda, cinnamon, ginger, cloves, and salt with a wire whisk. Add the flour mixture to the shortening mixture, and mix until combined. Chill the dough in the refrigerator for 1 hour.

Preheat oven to 375°F, and line a baking sheet with parchment paper. Shape the dough into 1-inch balls using your hands. Dip each ball into the ½ cup of granulated sugar, and sprinkle a couple of drops of water onto each ball using your fingers. Place each ball on the baking sheet.

Bake for 12 to 14 minutes, or until lightly browned. Cool completely on the baking sheet.

Gingerbread Kids

Gingerbread cookies are an essential cookie to make during the holidays. These have a great but not too strong molasses flavor.

YIELD: 2 DOZEN COOKIES

½ cup dairy-free margarine

½ cup light brown sugar

½ cup molasses

¼ cup unsweetened applesauce

2¼ cups unbleached all-purpose flour

1 teaspoon baking soda

1 teaspoon ground ginger

1 teaspoon ground cinnamon

⅛ teaspoon ground cloves

⅛ teaspoon salt

In the bowl of a stand mixer fitted with the paddle attachment, combine the margarine with the brown sugar, molasses, and applesauce. In a separate medium bowl, combine the flour, baking soda, ginger, cinnamon, cloves, and salt with a wire whisk. Add the flour mixture to the margarine mixture, and mix on medium low for about 1 minute. Chill the dough in the refrigerator for at least 1 hour.

Preheat oven to 350°F, and line 2 baking sheets with parchment paper. Roll the dough to a ¼-inch thickness on a lightly floured board. Cut shapes out with cookie cutters dipped in flour, and place the shapes on the prepared baking sheets. Bake for 8 to 10 minutes, or until lightly browned. Cool completely on the baking sheets.

Easy Cookie Icing

1 cup confectioners' sugar, sifted

1 teaspoon vanilla extract

1–2 tablespoons soy or rice milk

Food coloring (optional)

In a small bowl, combine the confectioners' sugar, vanilla, and soy milk with a small wire whisk until combined. Add drops of food coloring, if desired.

Soy Nut Butter Cookies

Before I had a child with food allergies, I loved peanut butter. I loved PB and J sandwiches, peanut butter cookies, the list goes on. After John was diagnosed with a severe peanut allergy, I quickly realized I couldn't have any peanut butter in my house. I've since replaced my peanut butter addiction with a soy nut butter addiction. These cookies are my new favorite "peanut butter" cookie.

YIELD: 2 DOZEN COOKIES

½ cup dairy-free shortening (see page 15)

½ cup creamy soy nut butter

½ cup granulated sugar

½ cup brown sugar

¼ cup unsweetened applesauce

1½ cups unbleached all-purpose flour

½ teaspoon baking powder

¾ teaspoon baking soda

¼ teaspoon salt

In the bowl of a stand mixer fitted with the paddle attachment, thoroughly combine the shortening, soy nut butter, sugars, and applesauce. In a separate medium bowl, combine the flour, baking powder, baking soda, and salt with a wire whisk. Add the flour mixture to the shortening mixture, and stir until just combined. Chill the dough for 1 hour.

Preheat oven to 375°F, and line 2 baking sheets with parchment paper. Using your hands, shape the dough into 1-inch balls, and place the balls onto the baking sheets. Dip a fork into some flour, and press the fork tines into each dough ball twice, making a crisscross design. Bake for 12 to 14 minutes, or until light brown. Cool completely on the baking sheets.

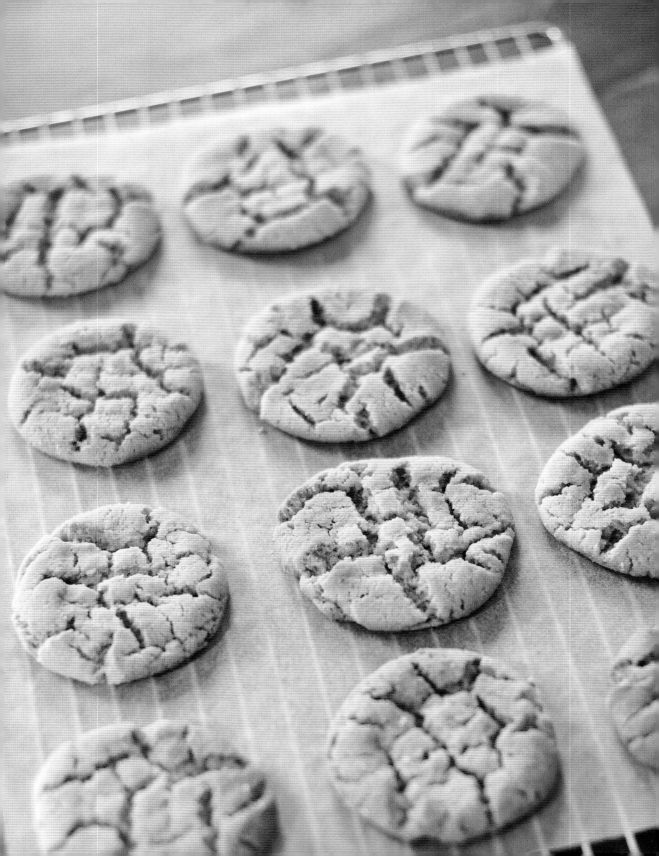

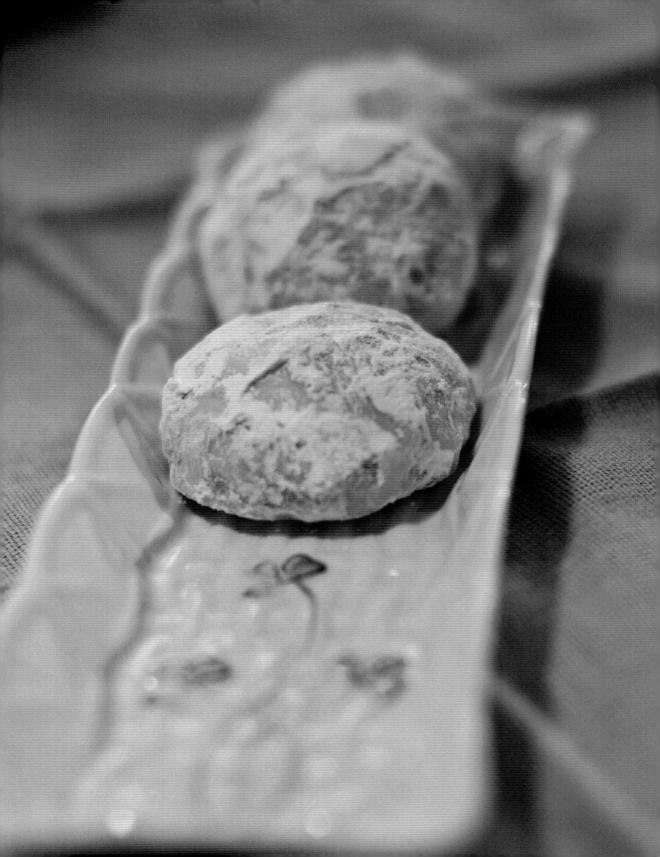

No-Nuts Russian Teacakes

Russian teacakes, which are also known as Mexican wedding cake cookies, are the cookies I always go looking for during the holidays. They are ridiculously simple to make, and no one will even notice the nuts are gone.

YIELD: 2 DOZEN COOKIES

1 cup dairy-free margarine

½ cup confectioners' sugar

1½ teaspoons vanilla extract

2¼ cups unbleached all-purpose flour

⅛ teaspoon salt

1 cup confectioners' sugar, for rolling

In the bowl of a stand mixer fitted with the paddle attachment, combine the margarine, the ½ cup sugar, and the vanilla until thoroughly combined. Stir in the flour and salt until the dough comes together into a pliable ball.

Preheat oven to 400°F, and line 2 baking sheets with parchment paper. Shape the dough into 1-inch balls, and place the balls onto the prepared baking sheets. Bake for 10 to 12 minutes, or until lightly browned. While the cookies are still warm but cool enough to handle, roll them in the remaining sugar. Cool completely, and roll in sugar again.

Chocolate Chip Bars

With four kids, I make a lot of treats for school functions, bake sales, parties, and holidays. If I need to make a big batch of something yummy in a hurry, this is the recipe I turn to. It is simple and fast, and it pleases kids and grownups alike. No one ever suspects it doesn't contain dairy, eggs, or nuts.

YIELD: 36 BARS

⅔ cup vegetable oil

1 cup unsweetened applesauce

3½ cups unbleached all-purpose flour

2 cups granulated sugar

3 teaspoons baking powder

¾ teaspoon salt

2 cups dairy-free chocolate chips

In a large bowl, combine the vegetable oil and applesauce. In a medium bowl, combine the flour, sugar, baking powder, and salt with a wire whisk. Add the flour mixture to the vegetable oil mixture, and mix well using a rubber spatula.

Preheat oven to 350°F, and spray a 15½×10½×1-inch jelly-roll pan with dairy-free baking spray. Stir in the chocolate chips, and spread the batter into the prepared baking pan. Bake for about 30 minutes, or until the top is light brown and an inserted cake tester comes out clean. Cool completely in the pan on a rack, and cut into small squares.

Chocolate Chip Brownies

It took me a long time to develop the perfect brownie recipe. It needed to have a nice balance of fudgy and cakey, and it had to taste like rich chocolate. I tested this recipe with neighborhood kids who don't have food allergies, and it was loved by everyone.

YIELD: 16 BARS

½ cup dairy-free shortening (see page 15)

1 cup granulated sugar

½ cup silken tofu

1 teaspoon vanilla extract

⅔ cup unbleached all-purpose flour

½ cup cocoa powder

½ teaspoon baking powder

¼ teaspoon salt

½ cup dairy-free mini chocolate chips

Confectioners' sugar, for dusting

In the bowl of a stand mixer fitted with the paddle attachment, thoroughly combine the shortening, granulated sugar, tofu, and vanilla. In a separate bowl, combine the flour, cocoa powder, baking powder, and salt with a wire whisk. Add the flour mixture to the shortening mixture, and mix until just combined. Stir in the chocolate chips with a rubber spatula.

Preheat oven to 350°F, and spray an 8-inch square baking dish with dairy-free baking spray. Spread the batter into the prepared baking pan, and bake for 30 minutes, or until an inserted cake tester comes out clean. Cool completely, and dust with confectioners' sugar.

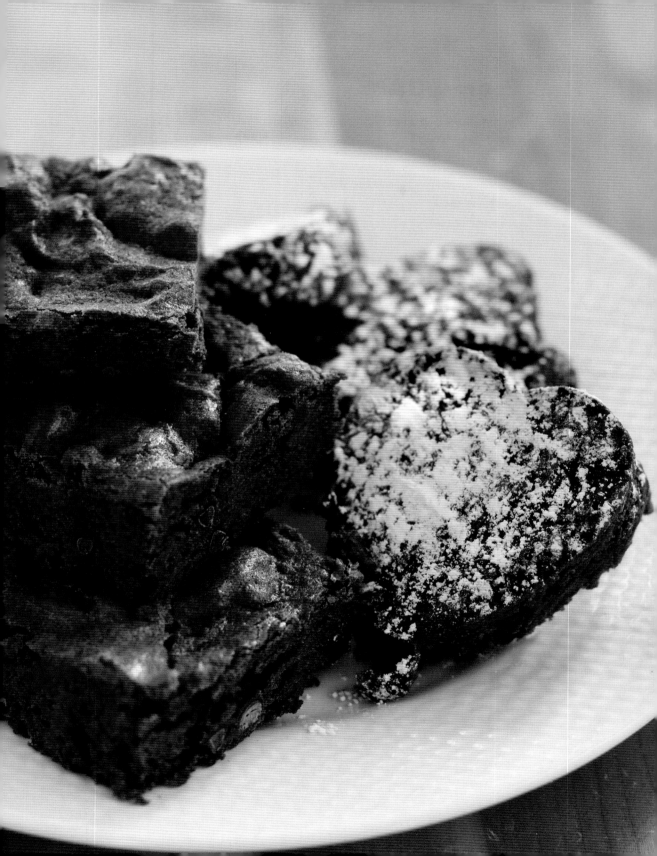

Raspberry Bars

I love cereal bars and wanted to create a bar that was similar in taste. These bars can be made with any type of jam you like.

YIELD: 36 BARS

½ cup dairy-free margarine, room temperature

1 cup light brown sugar

1½ cups unbleached all-purpose flour

½ teaspoon baking soda

¼ teaspoon salt

1½ cups quick-cooking oats

¼ cup water

2 cups raspberry or strawberry jam

1 teaspoon lemon juice

½ teaspoon grated lemon zest

In the bowl of a stand mixer fitted with the paddle attachment, cream together the margarine and sugar until light and fluffy. In a separate medium bowl, combine the flour, baking soda, and salt with a wire whisk. Add the flour mixture to the margarine mixture, and combine until the mixture is crumbly, scraping down the sides of the bowl as needed. Add the oats and water; mix with a rubber spatula until just combined.

Preheat oven to 350°F, and spray a 13×9-inch glass Pyrex baking dish with dairy-free baking spray. Combine the fruit jam with the lemon juice and zest in a small bowl and set aside.

Spread half of the batter into the prepared baking pan. Spread the jam mixture on top of the batter base. Add the remainder of the batter by sprinkling it evenly over the jam mixture. Bake for 25 to 30 minutes, or until set. Cool completely, and cut into bars.

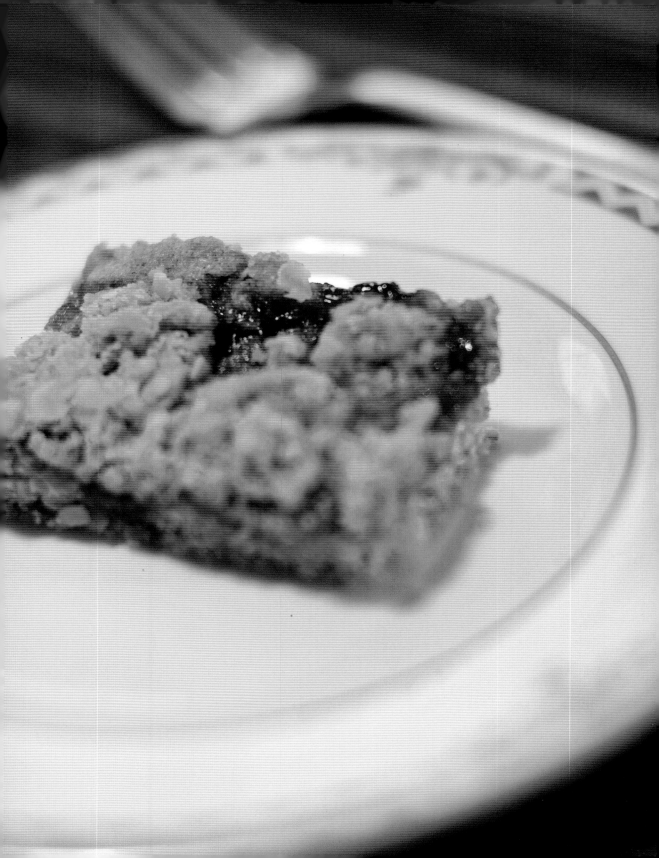

Cakes and Cupcakes

There is no other dessert that symbolizes celebration more than the cake. Many of our most important moments in life are celebrated with cakes and cupcakes. Whether it is your child's first birthday party or your wedding day, you probably served a favorite cake to mark the occasion.

I still have my mother's 13×9-inch glass Pyrex cake pan, the same one she used to bake birthday cakes for me and my five brothers and sisters. Her cakes were simple and straightforward, with hardly any fancy decoration. What we really loved about her cakes is that they were special—they were made just for us, and they made us feel loved and cared for.

These are some of my favorite cake recipes that I make for all my family's important celebrations. I also turn to the cupcake recipes for my son's class parties and birthday parties. Sometimes I make the cupcakes just because I want to surprise my kids with an extra-special after-school treat. I am confident that these cakes will become a part of your family's traditions, too.

Emerald Isle Coffee Cake

My mom, Jenness, had this coffee cake in her recipe box. She loved her sweets, and I inherited my passion for baking from her. An added bonus is the sweet cinnamon crumbs at the bottom of the cake.

YIELD: 1 CAKE

½ cup dairy-free margarine

1 cup granulated sugar

2 tablespoons water

1 cup dairy-free sour cream

1 teaspoon vanilla extract

2 cups unbleached all-purpose flour

1 teaspoon baking powder

1 teaspoon baking soda

1 teaspoon salt

1 recipe Cinnamon Filling (recipe follows)

Confectioners' sugar, for dusting

In the bowl of a stand mixer fitted with the paddle attachment, combine the margarine and sugar until light and fluffy. Add the water, dairy-free sour cream, and vanilla. Beat well.

Preheat oven to 350°F, and spray a Bundt pan with dairy-free baking spray. In a medium bowl, combine the flour, baking powder, baking soda, and salt with a wire whisk. Add the flour mixture to the margarine mixture, and beat well. Pour half of the batter into the prepared pan, and sprinkle the batter base with half the prepared recipe of Cinnamon Filling. Add the remaining batter, and top with the remaining Cinnamon Filling. Bake for 40 to 45 minutes, or until an inserted cake tester comes out clean. Cool completely, turn onto a serving plate, and dust with confectioners' sugar.

Cinnamon Filling

⅓ cup brown sugar

¼ cup granulated sugar

1 teaspoon ground cinnamon

In a small bowl, combine all ingredients. Mix well.

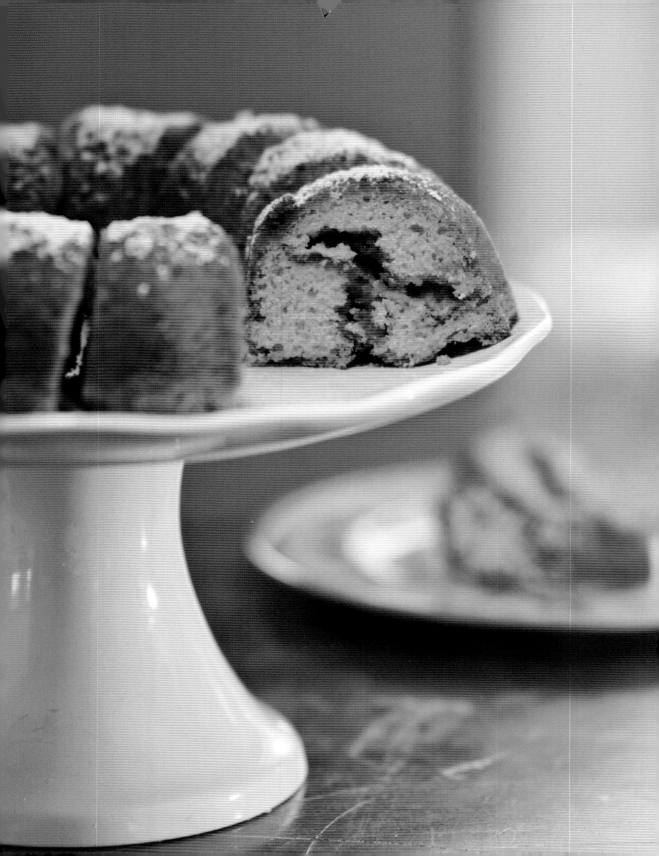

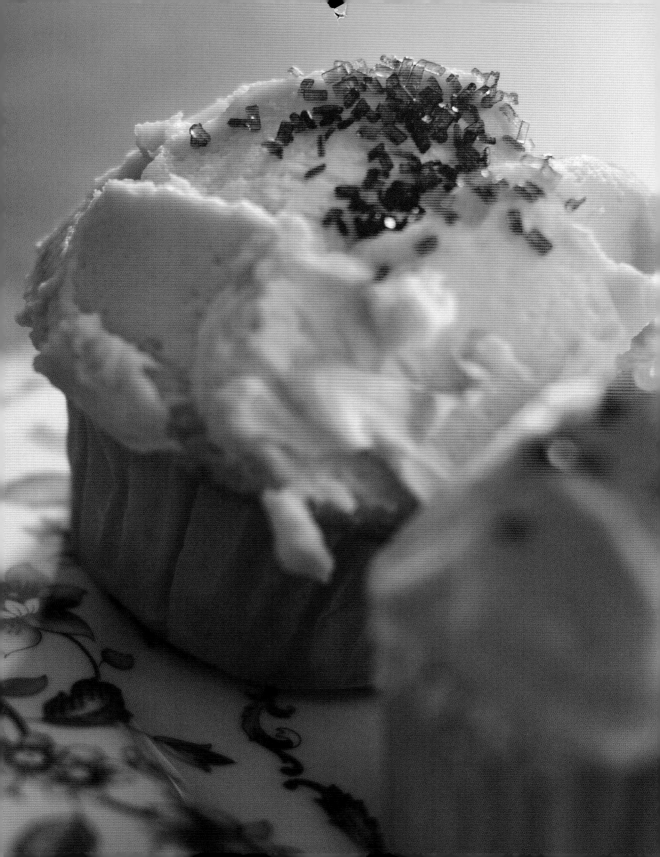

Classic Yellow Birthday Cake

I used to think yellow cakes lacked good flavor. This yellow cake is different. It is light and airy, too. The recipe makes a slightly smaller cake, so if you want a double-layer yellow cake, be sure to double the recipe.

YIELD: ONE 9-INCH SINGLE LAYER CAKE

½ cup dairy-free margarine

1 cup granulated sugar

1 cup soy milk

1 teaspoon vanilla extract

½ cup silken tofu

2 cups cake flour

2 teaspoons baking powder

½ teaspoon salt

In the bowl of a stand mixer fitted with the paddle attachment, combine the margarine and sugar until light and fluffy. Add the soy milk, vanilla, and tofu, and mix until thoroughly combined. In a separate medium bowl, combine the cake flour, baking powder, and salt with a wire whisk. Add the cake flour mixture to the margarine–soy milk mixture and mix on low for 1 minute until combined. Increase the speed to medium high and beat for an additional 3 to 4 minutes.

Preheat oven to 375°F, and generously spray one 9-inch cake pan or a 13×9-inch baking pan with dairy-free baking spray. Pour the batter into the prepared cake pan, and bake for 25 to 30 minutes, or until an inserted cake tester comes out clean. Cool completely before frosting.

Classic Yellow Cupcakes

Prepare the Classic Yellow Birthday Cake recipe as directed. Line 12 cupcake molds with paper liners. Pour the batter into the prepared pans, and bake for 20 to 25 minutes, or until an inserted cake tester comes out clean. Cool completely before frosting.

Classic Chocolate Birthday Cake

Early on in my son's life, I had to learn how to make a delicious cake for birthdays and parties. This recipe's batter can be used to make a 8-inch layer cake, a 13×9-inch rectangular cake, or a double batch of cupcakes. I still use the same 13×9-inch Pyrex pan my mother used to make our birthday cakes when I was a child.

YIELD: ONE 8-INCH LAYER CAKE OR ONE 13×9-INCH CAKE.

½ cup dairy-free shortening (see page 15)

1½ cups dairy-free buttermilk (1½ cups soy or rice milk mixed with 1½ tablespoons white vinegar; let it sit for 5–10 minutes)

2 tablespoons water

1 teaspoon vanilla extract

2 cups cake flour

1½ cups granulated sugar

⅔ cup cocoa powder

1½ teaspoons baking soda

½ teaspoon salt

Your choice of frosting (see pages 129–130)

In the bowl of a stand mixer fitted with the paddle attachment, combine the shortening, buttermilk, water, and vanilla until thoroughly mixed. In a separate medium bowl, combine the cake flour, sugar, cocoa powder, baking soda, and salt with a wire whisk. Slowly add the dry ingredients to the shortening mixture, and beat on high speed for 3 to 4 minutes, occasionally scraping the sides of the bowl with a rubber spatula.

Preheat oven to 350°F, and spray two 8-inch round cake pans or a 13×9-inch glass baking dish with dairy-free baking spray. Pour the batter into the prepared pans, and bake for 25 to 30 minutes, or until an inserted cake tester comes out clean. Cool completely before frosting.

Classic Chocolate Birthday Cupcakes

Prepare the Classic Chocolate Birthday Cake recipe as directed. Line 24 cupcake molds with paper liners. Pour the batter evenly into the liners, and bake for 20 to 25 minutes. Cool completely before frosting.

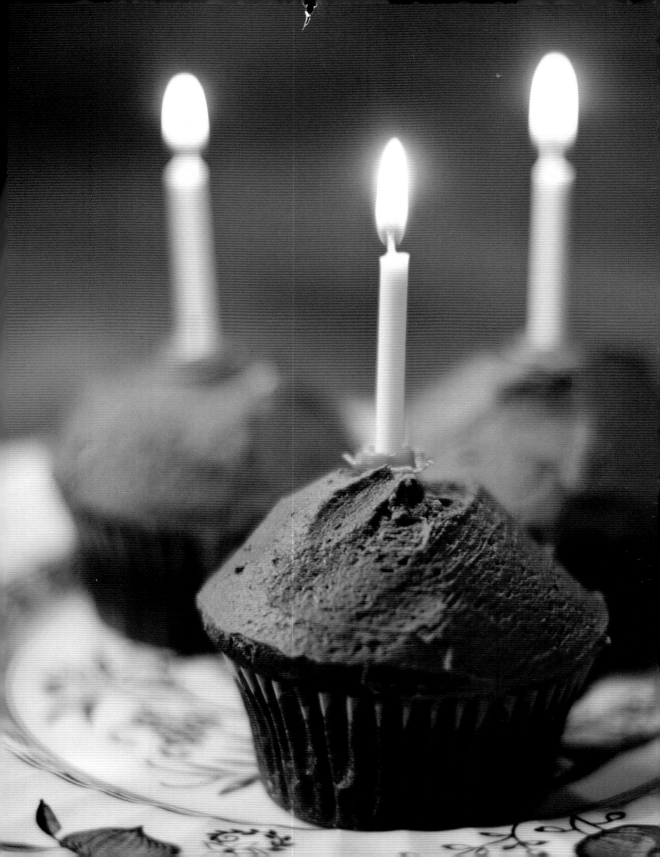

Classic Pound Cake

The original American version of the pound cake got its name from its heavy list of ingredients: a pound of eggs, a pound of butter, a pound of sugar, and a pound of flour. Obviously, the recipe came from someone who didn't have food allergies! This pound cake recipe is baked in a Bundt pan and uses silken tofu to give it the proper density. Make sure you purée the tofu in a blender first, because doing so will help it incorporate into the batter more evenly.

YIELD: 1 CAKE

1 cup dairy-free margarine

1¼ cups granulated sugar

1 cup silken tofu, puréed in a blender

2½ teaspoons vanilla extract

3 cups cake flour

½ teaspoon baking powder

½ teaspoon baking soda

½ teaspoon salt

1 cup dairy-free buttermilk (1 cup soy or rice milk mixed with 1 tablespoon white vinegar; let it sit for 5–10 minutes)

Icing (see page 129–130) or confectioners' sugar, for dusting

In the bowl of a stand mixer fitted with the paddle attachment, combine the margarine and sugar until light and fluffy. Add the silken tofu and vanilla slowly while the mixer is running at medium-low speed.

Preheat oven to 325°F, and spray a Bundt pan with dairy-free baking spray. In a separate medium bowl, combine the flour, baking powder, baking soda, and salt with a wire whisk. Add the flour mixture to the margarine mixture in batches, alternating the additions with the dairy-free buttermilk. Once all the ingredients are incorporated, mix on high for 3 minutes. Pour the batter into the prepared pan, and bake for 50 to 60 minutes, or until the top is golden brown and an inserted cake tester comes out clean. Cool the cake in the pan on a wire rack. Drizzle with icing or sprinkle with confectioners' sugar.

Gingerbread Cake

This is a simple and delicious cake that needs only a dusting of confectioners' sugar.

YIELD: 1 CAKE

½ cup dairy-free shortening (see page 15)

⅓ cup granulated sugar

¾ cup molasses

¾ cup plus 1 tablespoon hot water

2⅓ cups unbleached all-purpose flour

1½ teaspoons ground cinnamon

1 teaspoon ground ginger

1 teaspoon baking soda

¼ teaspoon salt

Confectioners' sugar, for dusting

Soy ice cream, for serving

In the bowl of a stand mixer fitted with the paddle attachment, combine the shortening, sugar, molasses, and hot water. In a separate medium bowl, combine the flour, cinnamon, ginger, baking soda, and salt with a wire whisk. Add to shortening mixture, and beat on medium-high for 2 to 3 minutes, scraping the bowl occasionally.

Preheat oven to 325°F, and spray an 8-inch glass baking dish with dairy-free baking spray. Pour the batter into the prepared pan, and bake for 40 to 50 minutes, or until an inserted cake tester comes out clean. Cool completely in pan, and serve dusted with confectioners' sugar and with soy ice cream.

Carrot Cake

This is one of our family's favorite cakes, hands down. It is the cake my daughter always requests for her birthday, and she doesn't even have food allergies. Make sure the cake is cooled and the frosting is chilled before icing the cake. Store, covered, in the refrigerator.

YIELD: 1 CAKE

1 cup granulated sugar

½ cup brown sugar

1 cup silken tofu

1 cup vegetable oil

2½ cups unbleached all-purpose flour

1½ teaspoons ground cinnamon

1¼ teaspoons baking powder

½ teaspoon ground nutmeg

1 teaspoon baking soda

½ teaspoon salt

1½ cups grated peeled carrots

Dairy-Free Cream Cheese Frosting (see page 130)

In the bowl of a stand mixer fitted with the paddle attachment, combine the sugars and tofu. Slowly add the oil, continuing to mix until thoroughly combined. In a separate medium bowl, combine the flour, cinnamon, baking powder, nutmeg, baking soda, and salt with a wire whisk. Add in ½-cup batches to the tofu mixture, and mix on medium low. Stir in the carrots using a rubber spatula.

Preheat oven to 350°F, and spray a 13×9-inch baking dish with dairy-free baking spray. Pour the batter into the prepared pan and bake for 35 to 40 minutes, or until an inserted cake tester comes out clean. Cool completely, and frost with Dairy-Free Cream Cheese Frosting.

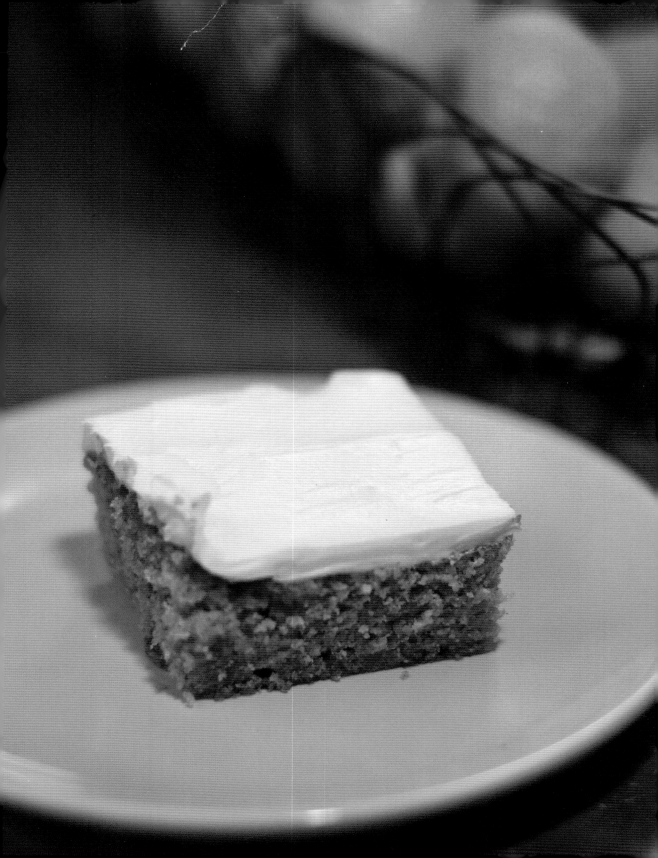

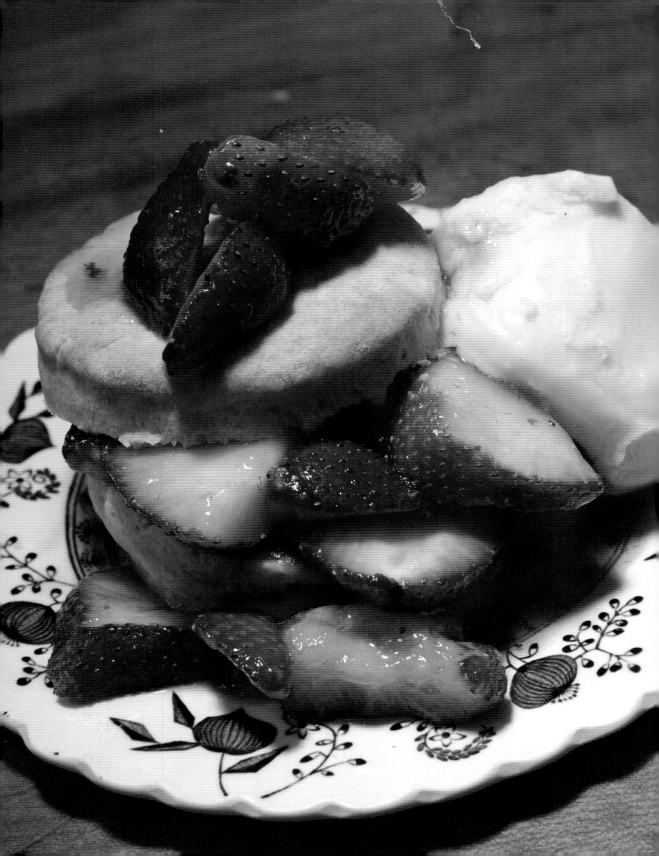

Strawberry Shortcake with Soy Ice Cream

I once went through a phase when all I wanted for dessert was strawberry shortcake. I'd look for it on the menu whenever my husband and I would go out to dinner. I had to make this for my kids because it has everything they love—strawberries, biscuits, and, instead of whipped cream, soy ice cream.

YIELD: MAKES 6 SHORTCAKES

4 cups fresh strawberries, hulled and sliced

½ cup granulated sugar

2 cups all-purpose flour

2 tablespoons granulated sugar

3 teaspoons baking powder

¼ teaspoon salt

⅓ cup cold dairy-free shortening (see page 15), cut into small cubes

¾ cup soy or rice milk

Soy ice cream, for serving

In a medium nonreactive bowl, combine the strawberries and sugar. Macerate at room temperature for 30 minutes. Set aside.

In a medium bowl, combine the flour, sugar, baking powder, and salt with a wire whisk. Using a pastry blender or your fingers, cut in the cold shortening until the mixture resembles coarse meal. Add the soy milk, and stir until just combined. Do not overmix.

Preheat oven to 425°F, and line a baking sheet with parchment paper. Shape the dough into a ball, and transfer to a lightly floured board. Knead the ball for about 5 minutes, and then roll it out into a ½-inch-thick disk. Cut out each shortcake with a floured 3-inch round cutter, and place the rounds on the prepared baking sheet. Bake until golden brown, 12 to 15 minutes. Cool slightly, and slice crosswise.

Place half of each shortcake biscuit on 6 plates. Fill each with the soy ice cream and ¼ cup of the macerated strawberries. Top with the remaining shortcake halves, soy ice cream, and an additional ¼ cup strawberries each.

Blueberry Buckle

This is another excuse for me to serve vanilla dairy-free soy ice cream with a yummy cake. It is a simple cake loaded with fresh fruit and topped with a crunchy streusel topping. You could substitute another fruit for the blueberries if you wish.

YIELD: 1 CAKE

½ cup dairy-free shortening (see page 15)

½ cup granulated sugar

1 tablespoon water

2 cups unbleached all-purpose flour

2½ teaspoons baking powder

¼ teaspoon salt

½ cup soy or rice milk

2 teaspoons freshly squeezed lemon juice

1 teaspoon grated lemon zest

½ cup blueberries (fresh or frozen)

Crumb Topping (recipe follows)

Soy ice cream, for topping

In the bowl of a stand mixer fitted with the paddle attachment, cream together shortening and sugar until light and fluffy. Add the water, and mix until combined.

Preheat oven to 350°F, and spray a 9-inch baking dish with dairy-free baking spray. Set aside. In a medium bowl, combine the flour, baking powder, and salt with a wire whisk. Add the flour mixture to the shortening mixture, alternating the additions with the soy milk, and beat well. Pour the batter into the prepared dish.

Combine the lemon juice, lemon zest, and blueberries in a small bowl. Sprinkle the blueberry mixture evenly over the batter in the dish, and top with the Crumb Topping. Bake for 50 to 60 minutes, or until an inserted cake tester comes out clean. Serve warm, with the soy ice cream.

Crumb Topping

½ cup flour

½ cup sugar

1 teaspoon ground cinnamon

¼ cup dairy-free margarine, cut into small pieces

Mix together all the ingredients, except the margarine, in a small bowl. Cut in the margarine with your fingers.

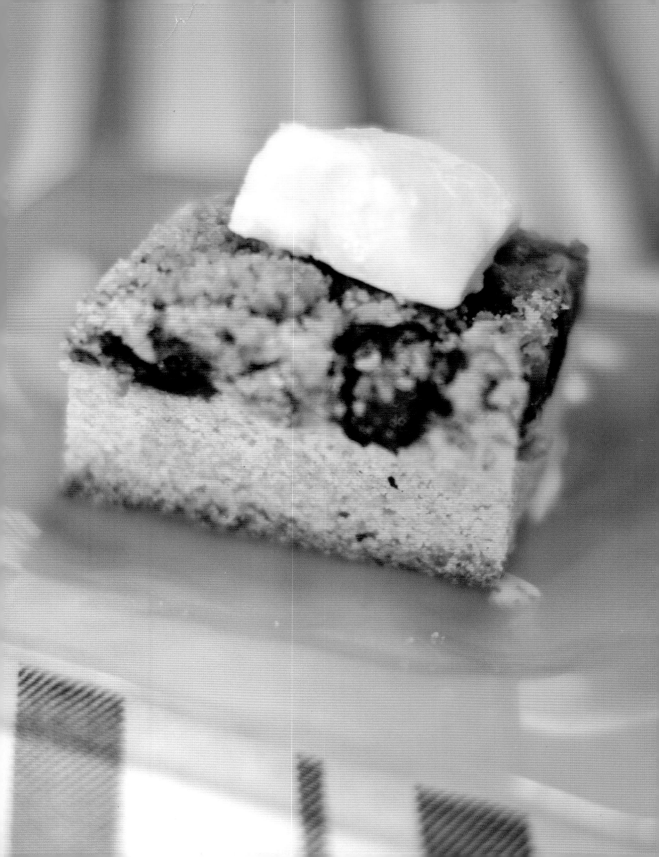

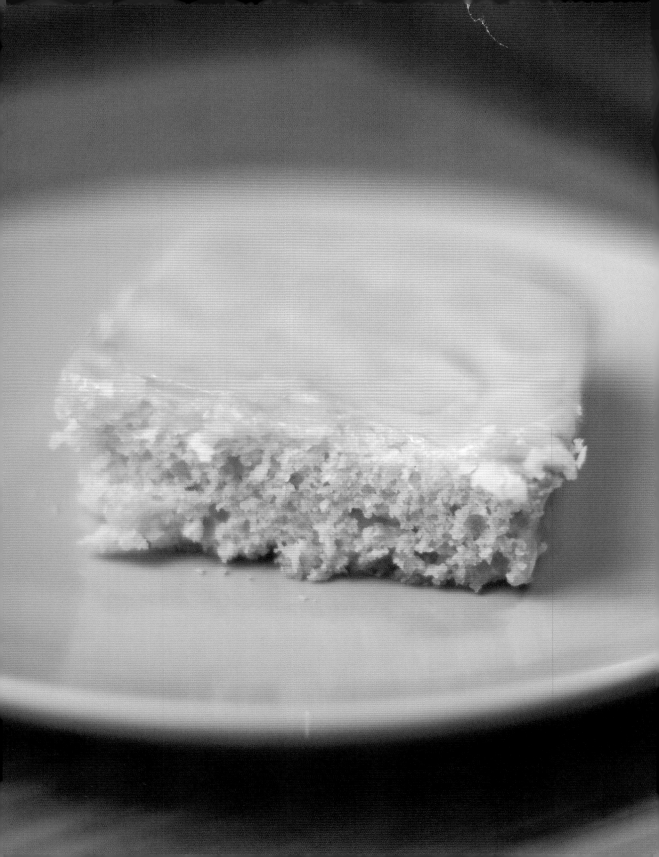

Lemon Cake

This is a simple little cake that can be dressed up, with Icing (see pages 129–130) and fresh berries, or dressed down, with just a good dusting of confectioners' sugar. It is perfect to serve for any special occasion, or when you just want to have something a little sweet.

YIELD: 1 CAKE

Cake

½ cup dairy-free margarine

1½ cups granulated sugar

1 teaspoon grated lemon zest

¾ cup silken tofu

2½ cups unbleached all-purpose flour

½ teaspoon baking soda

¼ teaspoon salt

½ cup soy or rice milk

¼ cup freshly squeezed lemon juice

Creamy Glaze

2 cups confectioners' sugar

1 teaspoon grated lemon zest

½ teaspoon vanilla extract

3–4 teaspoons soy or rice milk

In the bowl of a stand mixer fitted with the paddle attachment, combine the margarine and granulated sugar until light and fluffy. Add the 1 teaspoon lemon zest and the tofu, and beat well. In a separate medium bowl, combine the flour, baking soda, and salt with a wire whisk. Add the flour mixture to the margarine mixture, alternating the additions with the soy milk, and beat well. Stir in the lemon juice.

Preheat oven to 350°F, and spray a 13×9-inch baking dish with dairy-free baking spray. Set aside. Transfer the batter to the prepared baking dish, and bake for 25 to 30 minutes, or until an inserted cake tester comes out clean. Cool completely.

Combine the creamy glaze ingredients in a small bowl, and drizzle the glaze over the cooled cake.

Texas Sheet Cake

This is a large and delicious chocolate cake with a unique taste. Some old cookbooks say the cake got its name because the cake is as big as the state of Texas.

YIELD: 1 CAKE

¼ cup cocoa powder

1 cup dairy-free margarine

1 cup water

2 cups granulated sugar

2 cups unbleached all-purpose flour

1 teaspoon baking soda

2 tablespoons water

½ cup dairy-free buttermilk (½ cup soy or rice milk mixed with 1 teaspoon white vinegar; let it sit for 5–10 minutes)

1 teaspoon vanilla extract

Texas Glaze (recipe follows)

In a medium saucepan, bring the cocoa powder, margarine, and 1 cup water to a boil, stirring constantly over medium heat.

In a large bowl, mix together the sugar and flour. Pour the cocoa mixture over the sugar–flour mixture, and blend well. Add the baking soda, 2 tablespoons water, buttermilk, and vanilla.

Preheat oven to 400°F. Spray a 15×10×1-inch jelly-roll pan with dairy-free baking spray. Spread the batter evenly into the prepared pan, and bake for 20 minutes. While the cake is baking, prepare the Texas Glaze.

When the cake is done, immediately pour the Texas Glaze over it, spreading evenly.

Texas Glaze

½ cup dairy-free margarine

6 tablespoons soy or rice milk

4 tablespoons cocoa powder

1 teaspoon good-quality vanilla extract

2 cups confectioners' sugar

In a medium saucepan, combine the margarine, soy milk, and cocoa powder, and bring to a boil, stirring constantly. Remove from heat, and add the vanilla and confectioners' sugar; mix well. Immediately pour the glaze over the warm cake.

Farmer's Market Cherry Cake

This is delicious sprinkled with confectioners' sugar and served with a dollop of soy ice cream or all by itself. It is best when you can use the fabulous fresh cherries at your local farmer's market in the summer.

YIELD: ONE 9-INCH CAKE

1½ cups unbleached all-purpose flour

1½ teaspoons baking powder

⅛ teaspoon salt

½ cup silken tofu

¾ cup granulated sugar

½ cup dairy-free margarine, melted and cooled to room temperature

⅓ cup soy or rice milk

1 teaspoon vanilla extract

1 tablespoon lemon juice

2 teaspoons grated lemon zest

1 pint fresh cherries, rinsed and pitted

In a medium bowl, combine the flour, baking powder, and salt with a wire whisk, and set aside.

In the bowl of a stand mixer fitted with the paddle attachment, combine the tofu and sugar on medium-high speed until light and fluffy, about 2 minutes. Add the margarine, soy milk, vanilla, lemon juice, and lemon zest, and mix well. Add the flour mixture, stirring with a spatula until just combined. Lightly fold in the cherries.

Preheat oven to 400°F, and spray a 9-inch springform pan with dairy-free baking spray. Transfer the batter to the prepared pan, and bake for 10 minutes. Remove the pan from the oven. Bake for an additional 25 minutes, or until light golden brown and an inserted cake tester comes out clean. Cool completely on a wire rack.

Harvest Pumpkin Cake

I have a bit of an obsession with pumpkin-flavored treats. This one really takes the cake, pun intended! It is a beautiful and moist cake that is frosted with a delicious dairy-free cream cheese frosting.

YIELD: ONE 9-INCH LAYER CAKE

½ cup dairy-free shortening (see page 15)

1 cup granulated sugar

1 cup light brown sugar

½ cup silken tofu

1 (15-ounce) can pumpkin purée (not pumpkin pie filling)

2 teaspoons vanilla extract

3 cups cake flour

4 teaspoons baking powder

½ teaspoon baking soda

½ teaspoon salt

½ cup soy or rice milk

Dairy-Free Cream Cheese Frosting (see page 130)

In the bowl of a stand mixer fitted with the paddle attachment, combine the shortening, sugars, tofu, pumpkin, and vanilla extract on low speed until creamy. In a separate medium bowl, combine the flour, baking powder, baking soda, and salt with a wire whisk.

Preheat oven to 350°F, and spray two 9-inch round cake pans with dairy-free baking spray. Add the flour mixture to the shortening mixture, alternating the additions with the soy milk, and beat well. Pour into the prepared pans, and bake for 25 to 35 minutes. Cool completely, and frost with Dairy-Free Cream Cheese Frosting.

Dairy-Free Classic Cheesecake

Cheesecake can be tricky to get right. It is notorious for cracking and getting over- or under-baked. This allergen-friendly cheesecake is not only foolproof, but it's also utterly delicious.

YIELD: 1 CAKE

Easy Graham Cracker Crust (see page 134)

4 (8-ounce) packages Tofutti Dairy-Free Cream Cheese

1 cup granulated sugar

1 cup silken tofu, puréed in blender

1 packet gelatin

2 tablespoons fresh lemon juice

1 teaspoon grated lemon zest

1 teaspoon vanilla extract

Preheat oven to 350°F, and spray a 9-inch springform pan with dairy-free baking spray. Prepare the Easy Graham Cracker Crust recipe. Press the mixture into the prepared springform pan, and bake for 8 to 10 minutes, until set and lightly browned. Cool. Reduce oven temperature to 325°F.

Meanwhile, in the bowl of a stand mixer fitted with the paddle attachment, cream the dairy-free cream cheese until smooth. Scrape down the sides of the bowl with a rubber spatula, and add the sugar. Mix on low for a few seconds, until combined. With the mixer still running on low, slowly add the puréed tofu in a steady stream, mixing until thoroughly combined.

Mix together the gelatin and lemon juice in a microwavable bowl, and microwave for about 20 seconds, or until the gelatin is dissolved. Add the gelatin–lemon juice mixture to the cream cheese mixture, and mix on low for about 30 seconds. Add the lemon zest and vanilla, and stir just until combined.

Wrap the bottom of the prepared springform pan with aluminum foil, and place it in a jelly-roll pan. Fill the jelly-roll pan with warm water at a depth of ½ inch. Pour the cheesecake filling into the pan, and bake for about 1 hour, until the mixture is just set. (The center should jiggle a little.) Remove the pan and foil from the hot water, and cool completely on a wire rack. Cover with plastic wrap, and chill in the refrigerator overnight before serving.

Tip: It is important to make this cheesecake a day before you plan to serve it so it can chill overnight. This will ensure proper settling of the mixture.

Frostings and Icings

Don't bother to open a can of frosting. It's so easy to make your own and the result is worth it. Besides, many commercial frostings contain allergens. These fantastic basic frostings and icings are suitable for all your baking needs—the only frostings you'll need for everyday baking. Each recipe takes only about 5 minutes to whip up.

My Dairy-Free Cream Cheese Frosting tastes just as rich and creamy as the real deal, and it's perfect for my Harvest Pumpkin and Carrot Cakes (see pages 127 and 116). For a great all-purpose frosting on cupcakes and cakes, the Creamy Vanilla Frosting (see below) fits the bill (just a few drops of food coloring can make it virtually any color under the rainbow). My Creamy Chocolate Frosting (see page 130) is so light and airy that I have been known to eat it straight out of the bowl. Use it on either the Classic Chocolate or Classic Vanilla Cake (see pages 111 and 112). All of my frostings will stay fresh for a week if kept refrigerated in a tightly sealed container.

I also like to use my Classic Icing (see page 95) on my cookies, and it's also terrific as a simple glaze over a cake—try it with my Lemon Cake (see page 123). All you need to make it is a few ingredients, a small bowl, and a spoon—and maybe a few drops of color, if you are making icing for Cutout Sugar Cookies (see page 87) or Gingerbread Kids (see page 97). Let the kids mix it up, and drizzle away.

Creamy Vanilla Frosting

YIELD: 2 CUPS

1 cup dairy-free margarine

2 tablespoons soy milk

1½ teaspoons vanilla extract

⅛ teaspoon salt

2 cups confectioners' sugar

In the bowl of a stand mixer fitted with the paddle attachment, cream together the margarine, soy milk, vanilla, and salt until incorporated. Slowly add in the confectioners' sugar, and mix on low for 1 minute. Increase the speed to medium, and beat for 4 to 6 minutes, until light and fluffy. Chill about 30 minutes before using.

Dairy-Free Cream Cheese Frosting

YIELD: 2 CUPS

½ cup dairy-free margarine

¾ cup dairy-free cream cheese

⅛ teaspoon salt

1 teaspoon vanilla extract

2½ cups confectioners' sugar

In the bowl of a stand mixer fitted with the paddle attachment, cream together the margarine, cream cheese, salt, and vanilla until thoroughly combined. Slowly add in the confectioners' sugar, and mix on low for 1 minute. Increase the speed to medium, and beat 4 to 6 minutes, until light and fluffy. Chill about 30 minutes before using.

Creamy Chocolate Frosting

YIELD: 2 CUPS

1 cup dairy-free margarine

½ cup cocoa powder

¼ cup soy or rice milk

1 teaspoon vanilla extract

⅛ teaspoon salt

2 cups confectioners' sugar

In the bowl of a stand mixer fitted with the paddle attachment, cream together the margarine and cocoa powder until smooth. Add the soy milk, vanilla, and salt, and mix thoroughly. Slowly add in the confectioners' sugar, mixing on low for 1 minute. Increase the speed to medium, and beat 4 to 6 minutes, until light and fluffy.

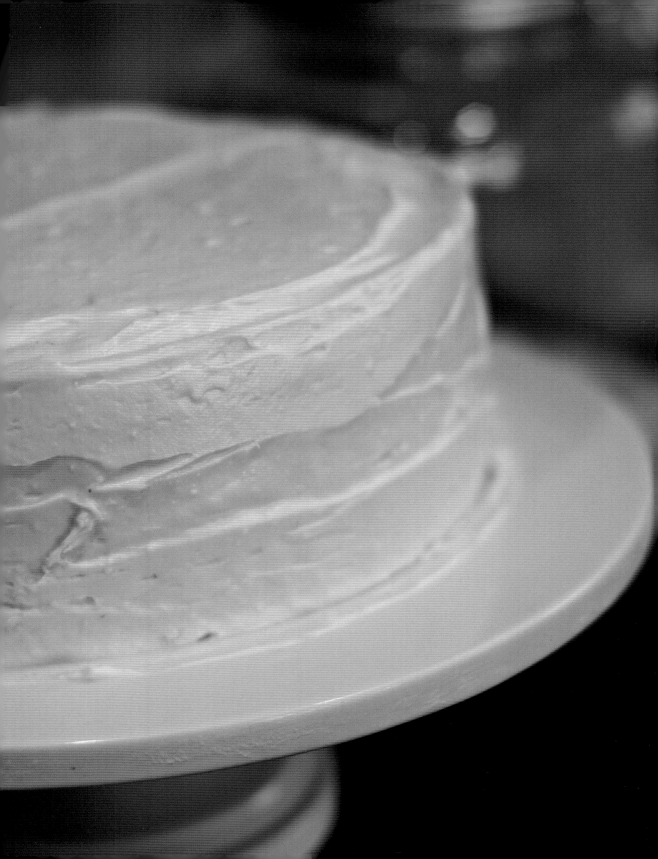

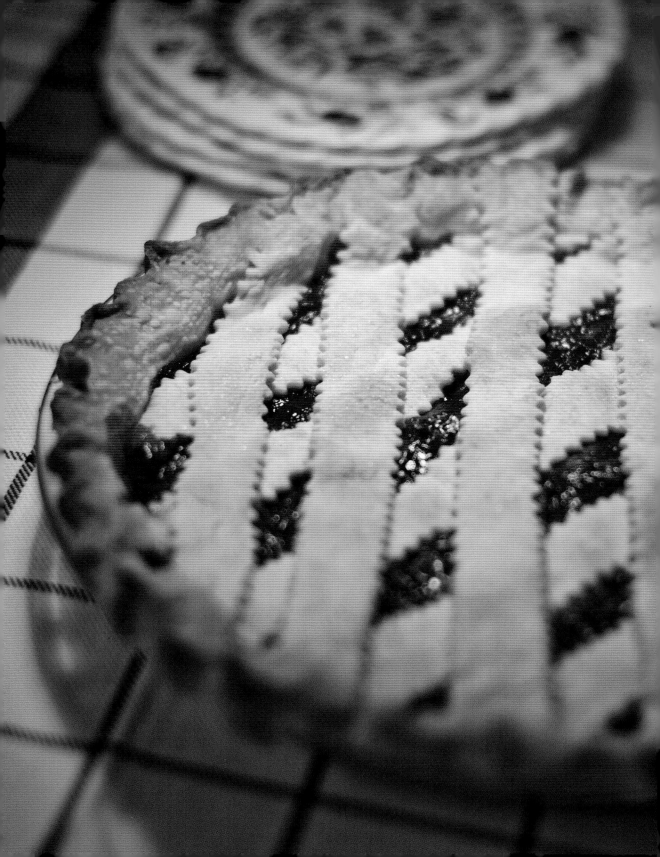

THE FOOD ALLERGY MAMA'S
Crisps, Pies, and Other Fruit Desserts

We have a family farm near Hayward, Wisconsin, that my husband loves to visit. On our first trip there together, we stopped at a diner in a small town that served what seemed like every type of pie imaginable. Since I have a deep affection for pies, I didn't even want to bother with lunch—I just wanted a cup of coffee and a few slices of pie to sample. My husband was skeptical, as he didn't think a lunch consisting of pie would hold me for the long road trip. Boy, was he wrong. I happily stuffed myself with apple, strawberry–rhubarb, chocolate silk, and summer berry pie until I was satisfied. For me, it was the highlight of the entire trip.

Pies are probably one of the most allergy-friendly desserts you can create. Make a great pie crust with dairy-free shortening (see page 15) and fill it with a variety of enticing options, such as Holiday Cranberry (see page 142), Door County Cherry (see page 145), or my personal favorite, Classic Apple (see page 141). There are no limits to what pie can do for you. It can soothe your soul and lift your spirits.

Traditionally, pies are a seasonal dessert, but my recipes can be made year-round. Buy lots of fresh berries, cherries, and apples when they are plentiful at the farmer's market, and freeze the extras you don't use right away in clearly labeled resealable plastic bags. Just reach in your freezer and make a beautiful pie any time—even in the dead of winter. Those same delicious frozen fruits can also be used for my Cherry Cobbler (see page 139) and Summer Berry Crisp (see page 151), and you don't even need to bother to defrost them. Cobblers and crisps are the perfect desserts to serve with dairy-free soy ice cream.

THE FOOD ALLERGY MAMA'S BAKING BOOK   **133**

Easy Pie Dough

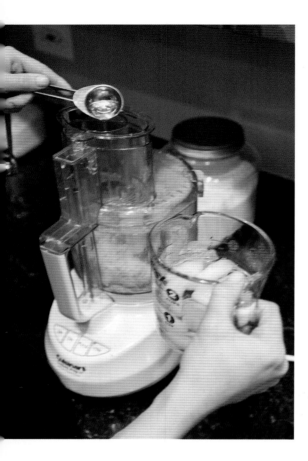

I've tried many pie-dough recipes over the years, but this is the version that never fails. Make sure your ingredients are all very cold, including the shortening. I keep Crisco Baking Sticks in the refrigerator specifically for making pie.

YIELD: MAKES ENOUGH DOUGH FOR A DOUBLE-CRUST 9-INCH PIE

2 cups unbleached all-purpose flour

1 teaspoon granulated sugar

½ teaspoon salt

⅔ cup dairy-free shortening (see page 15), chilled and cut into small pieces

5–7 tablespoons ice water

Combine the flour, sugar, and salt in the bowl of a food processor. Add the shortening, and pulse a few times until the mixture resembles small crumbs. Add the ice water, 1 tablespoon at a time, to the flour mixture, pulsing until the dough just comes together. Transfer the mixture to a sheet of plastic wrap. Use the plastic wrap to pull the sides of the dough together, forming a rounded disk. Chill for at least 30 minutes before using.

Easy Graham Cracker Crust

This is super easy to throw together, and a great base for my Cheesecake and Key Lime Pie recipes (see pages 128 and 146). Make sure your graham crackers are allergen free. I use Honey Maid Original Crackers.

YIELD: ONE 9-INCH PIE CRUST

1½ cups graham-cracker crumbs

¼ cup granulated sugar

5 tablespoons dairy-free margarine, melted

⅛ teaspoon salt

Preheat oven to 350°F. Combine all the ingredients in a medium bowl, and press the mixture into a 9-inch glass pie plate. Bake for about 10 minutes, or until the crust is set and lightly browned.

Summer Blueberry Pie

This is another delicious recipe to make after you've gone to the farmer's market and gotten plenty of summer's great bounty, the blueberry.

YIELD: 6 SERVINGS

Easy Pie Dough (see page 134)

6 cups fresh blueberries

¾ cup granulated sugar

3 tablespoons unbleached all-purpose flour

¾ teaspoon grated lemon zest

1 teaspoon fresh lemon juice

½ teaspoon ground cinnamon

⅛ teaspoon salt

1 tablespoon dairy-free margarine

Granulated sugar, for sprinkling

Prepare the Easy Pie Dough recipe as directed.

In a large bowl, combine the blueberries, sugar, flour, lemon zest. lemon juice, cinnamon, and salt, mixing with a rubber spatula.

Preheat oven to 400°F. Line the bottom of a 9-inch pie plate with half of the dough. Pour blueberry mixture into the pie shell, and dot the mixture with the margarine. Cover the blueberries with the remaining half of the dough, crimping the edges with your fingers. Cut three 1-inch slits on top of the dough, and sprinkle the pie with granulated sugar.

Bake for about 45 minutes, or until the fruit is bubbling and the crust is golden brown. Remove from the oven, and cool completely on a wire rack.

Apple and Cranberry Crumb Crostata

If you're pressed for time but want a fabulous fruit dessert, this is your best bet. Change the filling any way you want—pears, nectarines, mixed berries, and peaches would all be great here.

YIELD: 6–8 SERVINGS

Easy Pie Dough (see page 134)

2–3 Granny Smith apples, peeled, cored, and cut into 1-inch chunks

½ cup dried cranberries

1 teaspoon fresh lemon juice

½ teaspoon vanilla extract

¼ cup light brown sugar, divided

Soy ice cream, for serving

Prepare the Easy Pie Dough recipe as directed. Line a baking sheet with parchment paper. Preheat oven to 400 degrees. Transfer the dough disk onto the prepared baking sheet. Shape the dough into a 12-inch circle. Set aside.

In a medium bowl, combine the apples, cranberries, lemon juice, vanilla, and brown sugar. Place the apple–cranberry mixture on top of the dough, leaving a 2-inch border. Fold the dough gently toward the center, crimping as needed.

Bake for about 30 minutes, or until the dough is golden brown. Cool the crostata slightly on the baking sheet, and serve warm with the soy ice cream.

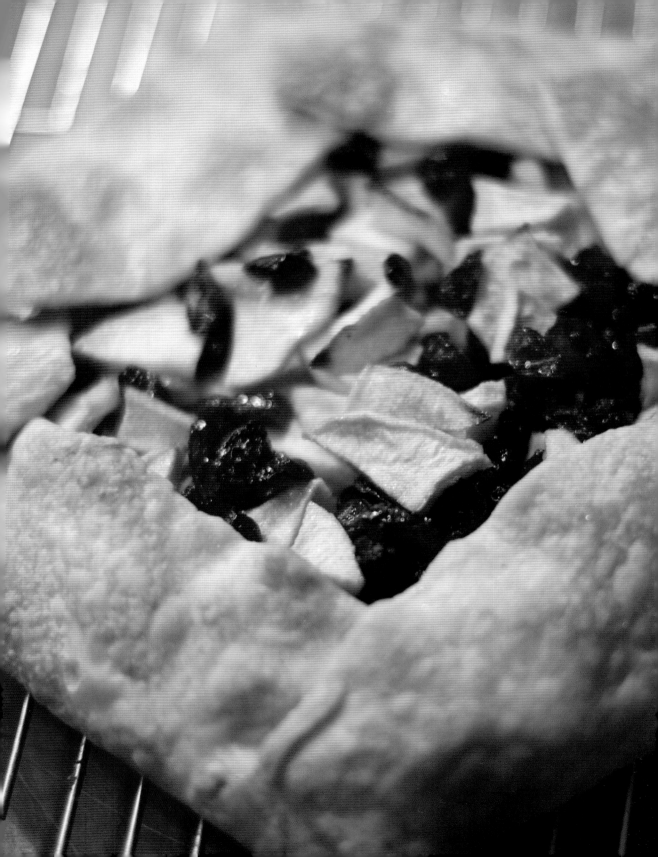

Classic Pumpkin Pie

Thanksgiving wouldn't be complete with a creamy pumpkin pie. This version is lighter than traditional versions made with evaporated milk and eggs. If you are short on time and want to use a store-bought crust, Pillsbury brand will do, as it doesn't contain any dairy or eggs.

YIELD: 6 SERVINGS

½ recipe Easy Pie Dough (see page 134)

1½ cups silken tofu, whipped in blender until creamy, divided

¾ cup packed light brown sugar

½ teaspoon vanilla

¼ teaspoon salt

1 teaspoon ground cinnamon

½ teaspoon ground ginger

½ teaspoon ground nutmeg

¼ teaspoon ground cloves

1 (15-ounce) can pumpkin purée (not pie filling)

Prepare the Easy Pie Dough recipe as directed. Preheat oven to 350°F. Fit the chilled pie dough into a 9-inch pie plate, and trim the dough to form a rim. Crimp the rim with your fingertips. Line the dough with aluminum foil, and place pie weights on top of the foil. Bake until the crust is very light brown, about 15 minutes.

Increase oven temperature to 425°F. In the bowl of a stand mixer fitted with the paddle attachment, combine ½ cup of the whipped tofu, the brown sugar, vanilla, salt, spices, and pumpkin. Add the remaining 1 cup whipped tofu, and beat well. Pour the mixture into the prepared pie plate, and bake for 15 minutes. Lower temperature to 350°F, and then bake for another 50 to 60 minutes, or until set. Cool to room temperature on a wire rack, and then refrigerate.

Cherry Cobbler

You could omit the frozen tart cherries here and use other fruits instead—perhaps blackberries and nectarines, or peaches and raspberries.

YIELD: 6 SERVINGS

1 cup granulated sugar

3 tablespoons cornstarch

¾ teaspoon ground cinnamon

4 cups tart cherries, pitted (can also substitute frozen tart or sweet cherries)

¼ teaspoon vanilla extract

1 cup unbleached all-purpose flour

1 tablespoon granulated sugar

1½ teaspoons baking powder

⅛ teaspoon salt

3 tablespoons dairy-free shortening (see page 15)

½ cup soy or rice milk

Soy ice cream, for serving

Preheat oven to 425°F, and lightly spray an 8-inch square glass baking dish.

In a medium saucepan, combine the 1 cup sugar, cornstarch, cinnamon, cherries, and vanilla over medium-low heat until the sugar is dissolved and the mixture is thickened and bubbling, about 2 minutes. Pour the cherry mixture into the prepared casserole dish, and set aside.

In a separate medium bowl, combine the flour, the 1 tablespoon sugar, baking powder, and salt with a wire whisk. Cut in the cold shortening with a pastry blender or your fingers until the mixture is crumbly. Stir in the soy milk, mixing until just combined.

Using a cookie scooper, scoop out 6 even portions of the flour mixture and drop them onto the hot fruit mixture.

Put the dish in the oven and bake for about 30 minutes, or until the biscuit topping is light golden brown and the fruit is bubbling. Serve warm, with the soy ice cream.

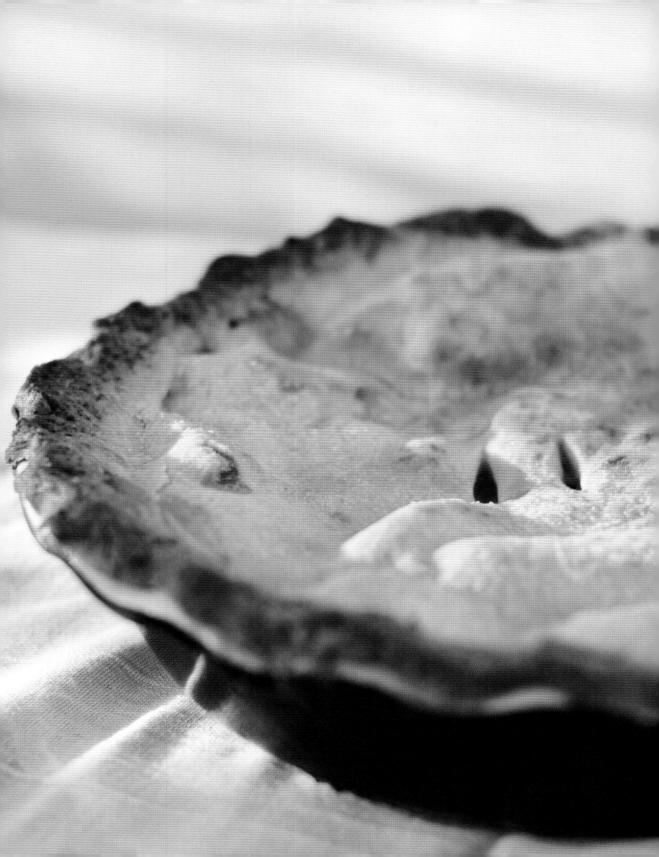

Classic Apple Pie

There's something so warm and comforting about a homemade apple pie. It's one of my favorite desserts.

YIELD: 6 SERVINGS

1 recipe Easy Pie Dough (see page 134), divided

1 cup granulated sugar

3 tablespoons unbleached all-purpose flour

1½ teaspoons ground cinnamon

¼ teaspoon ground nutmeg

¼ teaspoon salt

6½ cups apples (use a tart variety for best results), peeled, cored, and sliced into thick wedges

2 tablespoons dairy-free margarine, cut into small pieces

Granulated sugar, for sprinkling

Water, for sprinkling

Prepare the Easy Pie Dough recipe as directed. Split the recipe in half and set aside.

In a large bowl, combine the sugar, flour, cinnamon, nutmeg, and salt with a wire whisk. Add the apples, and mix well using a rubber spatula.

Preheat oven to 400°F. Line the bottom of a 9-inch pie plate with the dough, letting the dough hang over the sides. Fill with the apple mixture, and dot with pieces of margarine. Place the other dough round over the apples, and seal and flute the edges. Sprinkle the top of the pie with sugar and a few drops of water. Bake for 50 to 60 minutes, or until the apples are bubbling and the crust is lightly browned. Cover the edges with foil if the pie is browning too quickly.

Remove from the oven, and cool completely on a wire rack.

Holiday Cranberry Pie

The cranberry is a great little berry that injects lots of flavor and great color into any dish. This pie is not too sweet, and perfect for your holiday table. I love it served with vanilla soy ice cream.

YIELD: 6 SERVINGS

1 recipe Easy Pie Dough (see page 134)

1 cup water

1 tablespoon cornstarch

1½ cups granulated sugar

⅛ teaspoon salt

1½ teaspoons vanilla extract

1 cup raisins

2 cups fresh cranberries

2 teaspoons grated orange zest

Prepare the Easy Pie Dough recipe as directed and divide the dough in half. Set aside.

In a medium saucepan, heat the water and cornstarch until it boils and the cornstarch dissolves. Remove from heat, and add the sugar, salt, and vanilla. Cool to room temperature, and set aside.

Rinse the raisins in cold water to prevent sticking. Place the raisins and cranberries in the bowl of a food processor and pulse them a few times, just enough to roughly chop them. Add the raisins, cranberries, and orange zest to the cornstarch–sugar mixture, and mix well.

Preheat oven to 400°F. Line a 9-inch glass pie plate with the first rolled-out disk of pie dough. Pour the fruit mixture on top of the dough, and top it with the second rolled-out disk of dough. Crimp the edges, and bake for 10 minutes. Reduce oven temperature to 350°F, and bake for 25 to 30 more minutes, or until lightly browned and the fruit juices are bubbling. Cool completely.

Tip: Make sure to cool completely before serving, so this pie doesn't fall apart on you.

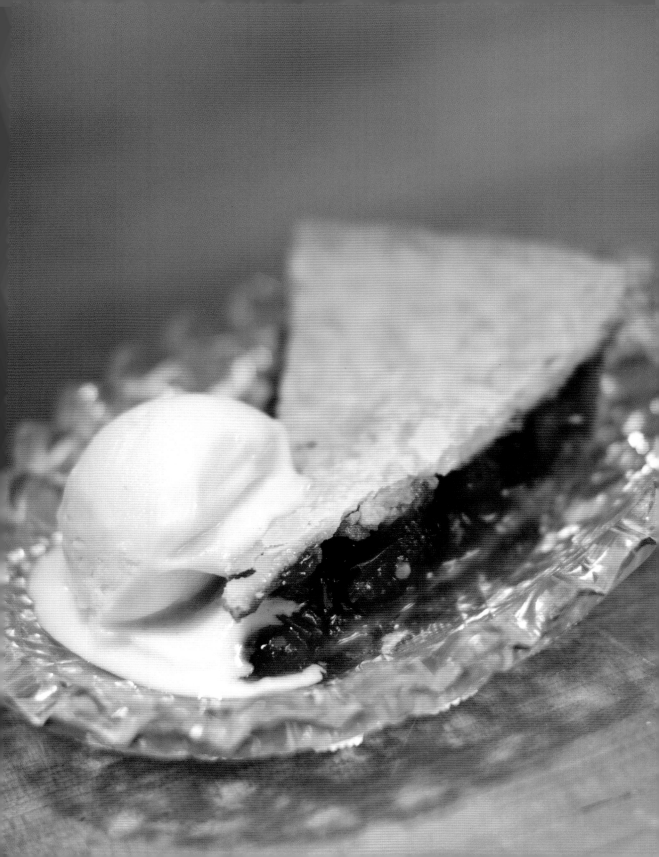

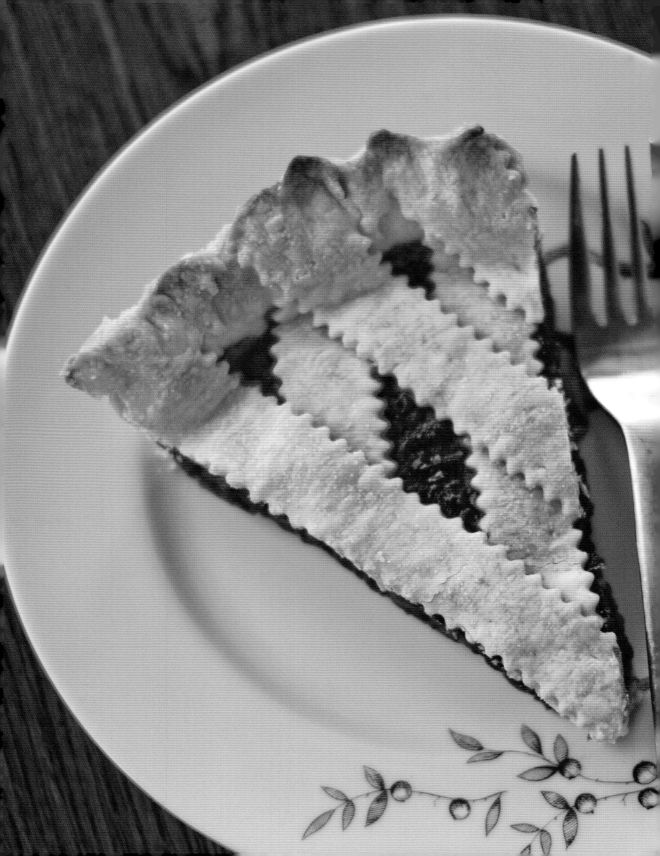

Door County Cherry Pie

My mother-in-law, Jeanne, makes this pie all year long using the fantastic tart cherries of Door County, Wisconsin. She gets them fresh during cherry season and freezes them in quart-sized freezer bags. Get in the habit of picking in-season fruit and freezing for later; your pies will thank you.

YIELD: 6 SERVINGS

1 recipe Easy Pie Dough (see page 134)

6 cups fresh or frozen red tart cherries, pitted (or 2 cans tart or sour pitted cherries, drained)

3 tablespoons cornstarch

¾ cup granulated sugar

¼ teaspoon vanilla extract

1 tablespoon dairy-free margarine, cut into pieces

Prepare the Easy Pie Dough recipe as directed, creating 2 disks of dough. Line a 9-inch pie plate with 1 rolled-out disk of dough. Set the second disk aside.

In a microwave-safe bowl, combine the cherries, cornstarch, and sugar, and microwave for 3 to 4 minutes, until thickened. Stir in the vanilla, and pour the cherry mixture into the prepared pie pan. Dot the top of the cherries with the margarine. Roll out the second disk of dough into a large (11-inch) rectangle. Cut the pastry into ½-inch strips, and weave the dough into a lattice design.

Preheat oven to 400°F. Bake for 35 to 40 minutes, until the fruit is bubbling and the crust is nicely browned. Cover the edges with foil if the crust is browning too quickly. Cool completely on a wire rack.

Tip: If you are using canned cherries, make sure they are thoroughly rinsed and drained. Add drops of red food coloring to restore the canned cherries' color to a vibrant red. You may also use frozen cherries.

Key Lime Pie

Key Lime Pie is one of those desserts our food-allergic children will never be able to order in a restaurant. I had to find a way to make a version that was as close to the real deal as possible. Let the pie sit in your fridge for a minimum of 4 to 6 hours before serving, and preferably overnight.

YIELD: 6 SERVINGS

1 recipe Graham Cracker Crust (see page 134), cooled completely

1 package silken tofu

1 (8-ounce) package Tofutti Dairy-Free Cream Cheese

½ cup plus 3 tablespoons fresh lime juice, divided

¼ cup granulated sugar

2 teaspoons grated lime zest

⅛ teaspoon salt

1 package unflavored gelatin

Prepare the Graham Cracker Crust recipe as directed.

In a blender, combine the tofu, cream cheese, ½ cup lime juice, sugar, lime zest, and salt until thoroughly puréed. In a small bowl, combine the gelatin and remaining lime juice, and microwave 20 seconds, until the gelatin is dissolved. Add the gelatin mixture to the blender, and mix thoroughly. Pour into the prepared Graham Cracker Crust, and chill at least 4 to 6 hours.

Note: It is very important to cool the prebaked pie crust completely before filling it. Otherwise, your graham cracker crust could get soggy while it sets up in the fridge.

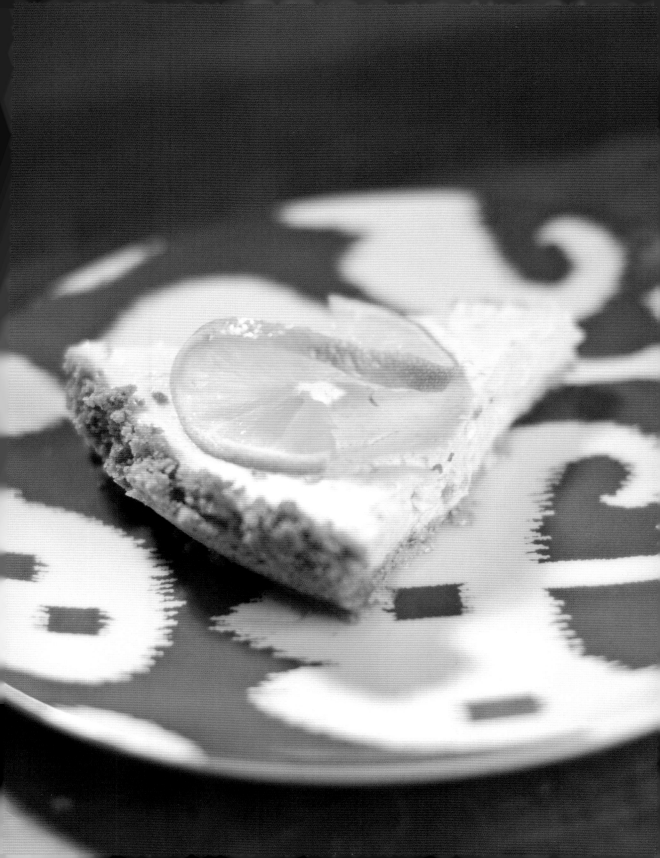

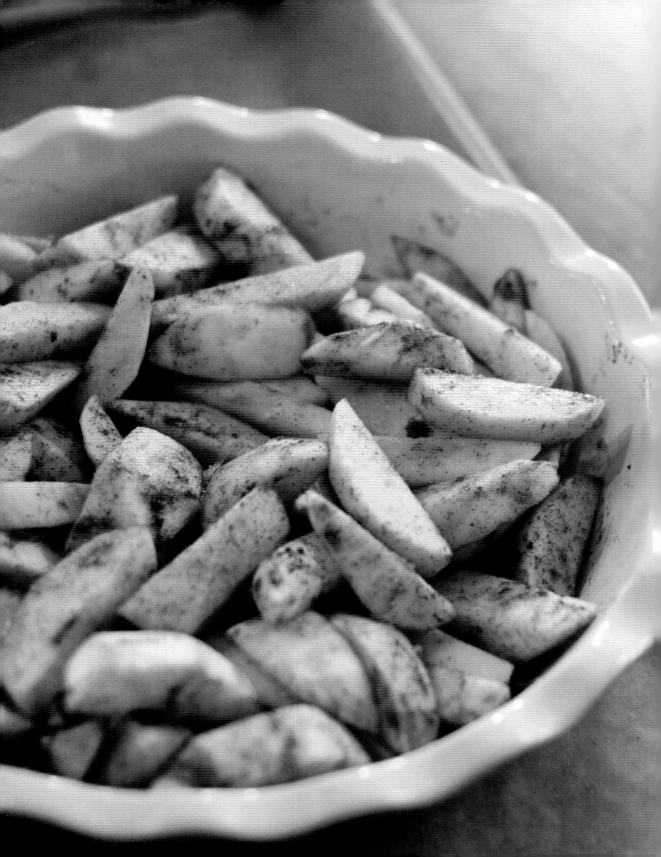

Apple Crisp

Apple crisp is the perfect fall dessert—warm, gooey, crunchy, and perfect with a scoop of soy ice cream. It's one of my top five desserts, and this particular recipe won rave reviews on my foodallergymama.com blog.

YIELD: 8–10 SERVINGS

Apple Filling

6–7 large apples, peeled and cut into 6 wedges

1 teaspoon grated lemon zest

2 teaspoons fresh lemon juice

⅓ cup granulated sugar

2½ teaspoons ground cinnamon

Crisp Topping

1 cup unbleached all-purpose flour

1 cup quick-cooking oats

½ cup light brown sugar

1 teaspoon ground cinnamon

⅛ teaspoon salt

½ cup dairy-free margarine, chilled and cut into small pieces

Spray an oval 14×9-inch casserole or 13×9-inch glass baking dish with dairy-free baking spray. Combine the apples with the lemon zest, lemon juice, sugar, and cinnamon in a large bowl, and pour the mixture into the prepared dish.

To make the topping, in a medium bowl, combine the flour, oats, brown sugar, cinnamon, and salt. Cut in the margarine using a pastry blender or your fingers. The mixture should clump into pea-sized pieces.

Preheat oven to 375°F. Sprinkle the crisp topping over the apples, and place the dish on a baking sheet. Bake for 50 to 60 minutes, or until the topping is golden brown and the fruit is bubbling.

Tip: Place the crisp on a baking sheet to catch any fruit that bubbles over.

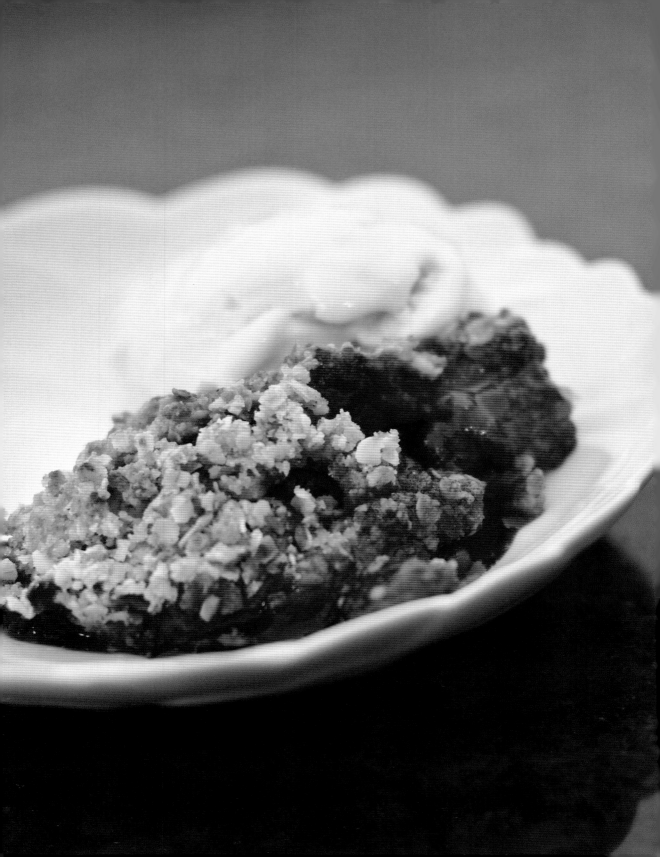

Summer Berry Crisp

I love fruit crisps and wanted to create a version that could be made all year long. You can use any assortment of frozen berries.

YIELD: 6 SERVINGS

Berry Filling

7 cups frozen mixed berries (blueberries, raspberries, and blackberries)

⅓ cup granulated sugar

1 tablespoon unbleached all-purpose flour

1 teaspoon fresh lemon juice

½ teaspoon grated lemon zest

Soy ice cream, for serving

Crisp Topping

1 cup old-fashioned oats

1 cup unbleached all-purpose flour

½ cup brown sugar

1 teaspoon ground cinnamon

½ cup dairy-free margarine, cut into small pieces

Preheat oven to 400°F. In a medium bowl, combine the berries, sugar, 1 tablespoon flour, lemon juice, and lemon zest. Place in an ungreased glass 8-inch square baking dish. Bake for 15 minutes.

To make the topping, in a medium bowl, combine the oats, 1 cup flour, brown sugar, and cinnamon with a wire whisk. Cut in the margarine using a pastry blender or your fingers. The mixture should clump into pea-sized pieces.

Take the fruit mixture out of the oven, sprinkle the crisp topping over it, and bake for about 30 minutes more, or until the fruit is bubbling and the crisp topping is browned. Serve the crisp warm, with soy ice cream.

Tip: There is no need to thaw the berries.

Italian Fruited Jam Tart

This is a traditional Italian dessert made with any variety of jam and topped with a decorative lattice weave. It looks and tastes elegant but is super simple.

YIELD: 8 SERVINGS

1¾ cups unbleached all-purpose flour

¼ cup granulated sugar

⅛ teaspoon salt

½ cup dairy-free margarine, chilled and cut into small pieces

2–4 tablespoons ice water

2 cups fruit jam (apricot, raspberry, strawberry, or blackberry)

2 tablespoons soy milk, for glaze

Combine the flour, sugar, and salt in a medium bowl. Cut the margarine into the flour using a pastry blender or your fingers. The mixture should be crumbly. Add the ice water, 1 tablespoon at a time, to the flour mixture until the dough just comes together. Shape the dough into a ball, wrap the ball in plastic wrap, and refrigerate for about 1 hour.

Divide the dough ball into two disks, one slightly larger than the other. Roll out the larger disk to a ½-inch thickness. Transfer the larger disk to a 9- or 10-inch tart pan that has been sprayed with dairy-free baking spray. Place the tart pan and dough in the refrigerator while you preheat the oven to 375°F.

Remove the tart dough from the refrigerator, and spread the jam evenly over the dough using an offset spatula. Roll out the remaining disk of dough, and cut the dough into strips about ½ inch wide. Weave the strips of dough into a lattice design. Trim the edges with a paring knife, and brush the lattice strips with the soy milk. Bake for about 30 minutes, or until the crust is a deep golden brown. Cool completely on a wire rack.

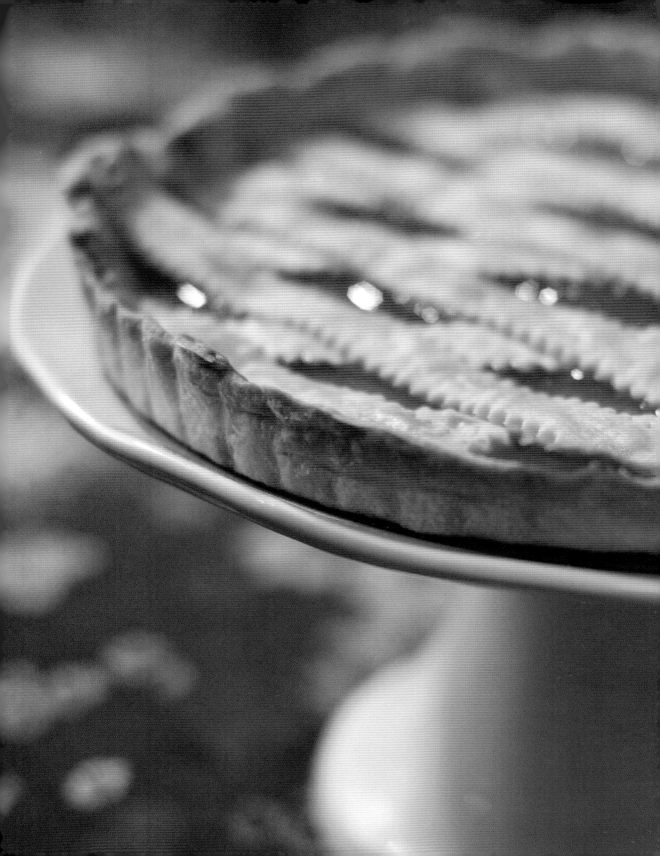

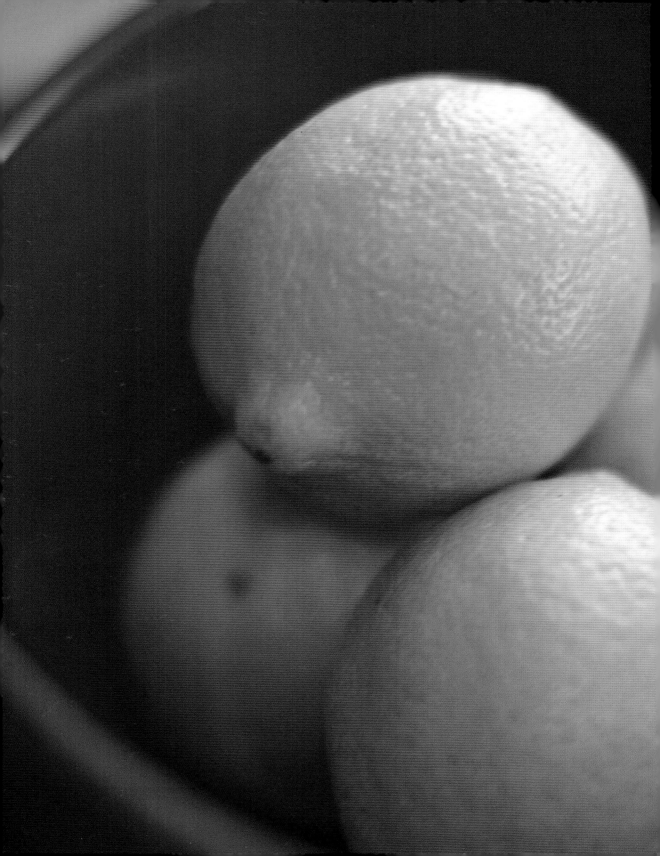

Other Sweet Treats

I'll bet you probably have a particular sweet treat that's positively necessary when you need a little pick-me-up. Treats like my Dairy-Free Chocolate Shake (see page 159), Lemon Granita (see page 156), and Caramel Corn (see page 162) are the perfect answer. These sweet treats make me happy no matter when I make them. The Lemon Granita is a fabulous dessert for a dinner party, the Chocolate–Soy Nut Butter Candies (see page 163) are special enough to give away as gifts during the holidays, and the Dairy-Free Chocolate Shakes (see page 159) are perfect anytime you want to make something simple but extra special.

These are also fun snacks to make with your children. My kids love to watch Hot Cocoa (see page 159) as it simmers on the stove on a cold winter day, and each of them gets to carefully stir the heavenly mixture with a whisk. Even the littlest children can participate when you make the Berry Breakfast Smoothie (see page 156), because nothing beats watching a blender do its magic when you're three years old.

No matter what treat you choose to make, be sure to make it with your children. They will love learning with you how something they're accustomed to seeing in a package, like Chocolate Caramel Corn (see page 162), can be made at home, or the ins and outs of making a perfectly fudgy treat, like my Snickeroos (see page 160). The best part is that all these recipes are dairy-, egg-, and nut-free and can be enjoyed by all—including children with food allergies.

Lemon Granita

My kids love this as a refreshing alternative to ice cream, but it is also elegant enough to serve at a dinner party in fancy fluted glasses. I pour the lemon–water mixture into an antique glass loaf dish. You could use any 8-inch loaf pan; cover it tightly with plastic wrap before putting it into the freezer.

YIELD: 6–8 SERVINGS

2 cups water

½ cup granulated sugar

2 teaspoons grated lemon zest

Juice of 2 lemons

In a small saucepan, combine the water and sugar, and heat on low until the sugar dissolves. Bring the mixture to a boil. Remove from heat, and cool to room temperature.

Add the lemon zest and lemon juice to the sugar syrup mixture. Cool to room temperature. Place the
mixture in a shallow glass container, and freeze until solid. Using a fork, scrape the lemon ice block into small crystals. Transfer the lemon ice crystals into serving glasses.

Berry Breakfast Smoothie

My littlest guys, David and Matthew, love *this breakfast smoothie. We make it often for an after-school snack, and it's a great treat for the kids to help with. I think the best part for them is hearing the loud blender rev its engine.*

YIELD: 4 SERVINGS

1 cup frozen strawberries

1 medium banana, sliced

1 cup dairy-free vanilla soy yogurt

1 cup orange juice

1 tablespoon honey

Put all the ingredients into a blender, and purée until smooth. Serve in tall glasses.

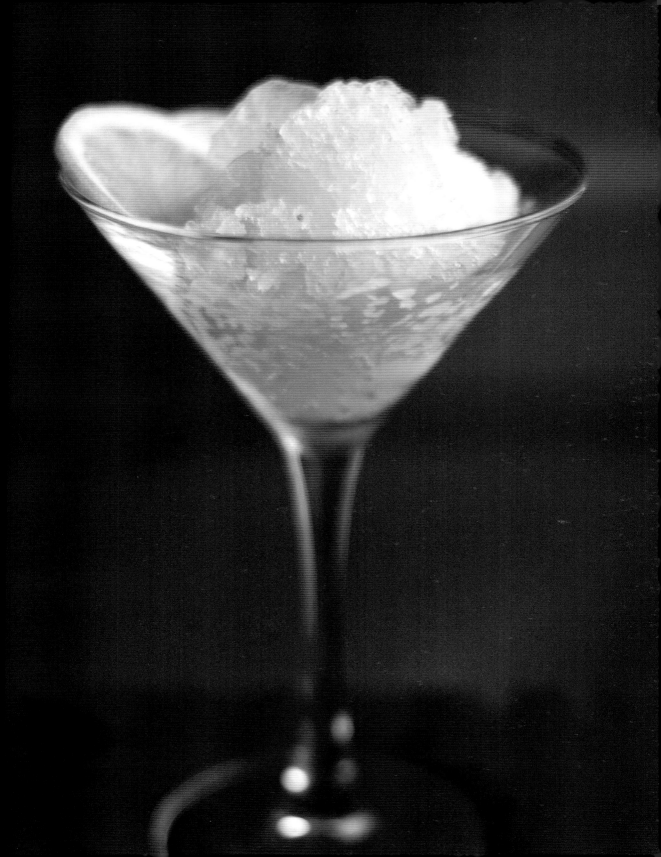

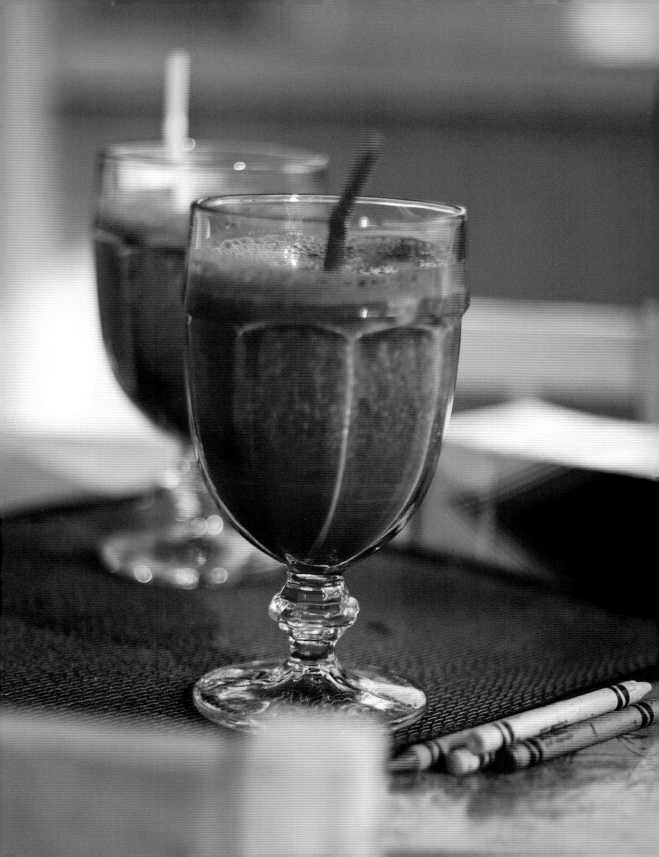

Dairy-Free Chocolate Shake

Children with food allergies can't order milkshakes from burger places and ice-cream shops. That's why I make this shake all the time at home. My children often request it when they are home sick from school.

YIELD: 2 SERVINGS

1⅓ cups soy or rice milk

½ cup dairy-free chocolate syrup

4–5 generous scoops vanilla soy ice cream

Combine the soy milk and chocolate syrup in a blender, and pulse for a few seconds. Add the soy ice cream and purée on low speed about 1 minute, or until the mixture is smooth and blended together. Serve in tall glasses.

Hot Cocoa

So many hot cocoa mixes on the market contain milk that I'd almost given up on making the concoction for my son. Then, it occurred to me that making my own hot cocoa from scratch would take no more than five minutes, so why not? Just the smell of hot cocoa simmering on the stove is worth the effort.

YIELD: 4 SERVINGS

⅓ cup unsweetened cocoa powder

⅓ cup granulated sugar

½ cup water

3¼ cups soy or rice milk

Large allergen-free marshmallows, for topping
(I use Kraft Jet-Puffed Marshmallows)

In a medium saucepan, whisk together the cocoa powder and sugar over medium-low heat. Stir in the water, and bring the mixture to a boil, stirring constantly. Add the soy milk. Reduce heat, and simmer for 5 minutes. Serve with the large allergen-free marshmallows.

Snickeroos

My mother-in-law, Jeanne, makes this decadent little treat with peanut butter, but I've made it peanut- and dairy-free. Kids go crazy for these little squares. Store Snickeroos in an airtight container.

YIELD: ABOUT 36 SQUARES

1 cup dark corn syrup

1 cup granulated sugar

1 (15-ounce) container creamy soy nut butter

6 cups crisped rice cereal

2 cups dairy-free chocolate chips

Spray a 13×9×2-inch baking pan generously with dairy-free baking spray. Set aside.

In a medium saucepan, boil the corn syrup and sugar together until the sugar is dissolved. Stir in the soy nut butter until thoroughly combined. In a large bowl, combine the cereal and the soy nut butter mixture, and press the batter into the prepared baking dish.

Place the chocolate chips into a microwavable dish, and heat on high 45 to 60 seconds, or until melted. Using an offset spatula, spread the melted chocolate over the batter. Let the mixture cool completely at room temperature, and cut into small 1-inch squares.

Tip: Add more rice cereal if you like a crunchier bar, and less cereal if you want your Snickeroos to be chewier.

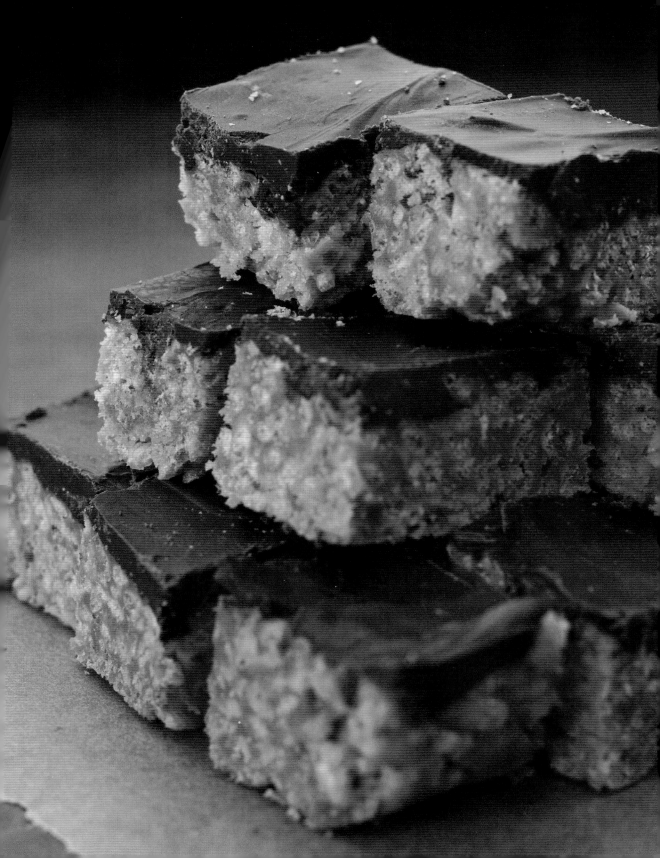

Caramel Corn

Caramel corn is another treat I just had to make in an allergen-free form for my kids. When John tried it for the first time, he loved it. Store at room temperature in a covered container.

YIELD: 4 SERVINGS

½ cup packed brown sugar

½ cup light corn syrup

¼ cup dairy-free margarine

6 cups popped corn

Line a baking sheet with parchment paper or a Silpat baking mat, and preheat oven to 325°F.

In a large, heavy pot, heat the brown sugar, corn syrup, and margarine over medium heat until melted. Add the popped corn, and stir thoroughly to coat. Remove from heat, and transfer to the prepared baking sheet. Bake the caramel corn for about 30 minutes, or until the caramel begins to set on the bottom. Remove from the oven and let cool. Break the caramel corn into clusters and store in resealable bags for up to 1 week.

Chocolate Caramel Corn

A yummy update to the classic version.

YIELD: 4 SERVINGS

1 cup dairy-free chocolate chips

1 recipe prepared Caramel Corn (see previous recipe), spread on parchment-lined baking sheet

In a microwavable bowl, heat the chocolate chips for 30 to 45 seconds, or until melted. Drizzle the melted chocolate over the caramel corn. Let the chocolate set completely, and then break the caramel corn into clusters.

Chocolate–Soy Nut Butter Candies

Every Christmas, my sister-in-law Vira brings her famous platter of cookies for dessert. Yes, it is a food-allergy nightmare, but her peanut-butter balls were so special and yummy, I had to make a peanut-free version using soy nut butter and dairy-free chocolate chips.

YIELD: ABOUT EIGHTY 1-INCH BALLS

3 sticks dairy-free margarine

1 teaspoon vanilla extract

2 (15-ounce) containers soy nut butter

5½–6 cups confectioners' sugar

3 (10-ounce) packages dairy-free chocolate chips

Line 3 large baking sheets with parchment paper.

In the bowl of a stand mixer fitted with the paddle attachment, combine the margarine, vanilla, and soy nut butter until creamy. Mix in the confectioners' sugar, 1 cup at a time, on low, scraping down the sides of the bowl as needed, until all the sugar is incorporated and the dough is soft and not too sticky. Form the dough into a large disk wrapped in plastic wrap, and chill the disk in the freezer for 10 minutes. Transfer the disk onto a floured surface, and knead lightly, about 15 times.

Place the chocolate chips into a large microwavable container and heat until melted, 30 to 40 seconds. Set aside for dipping.

Roll the dough into 1-inch balls. If the dough gets too warm, put the remainder back into the freezer to firm it up. Using a fork, coat the soy nut butter balls with the melted chocolate. Place the balls on the parchment paper to set. Repeat with the remainder of the dough. After all the balls have set, serve in paper candy cups.

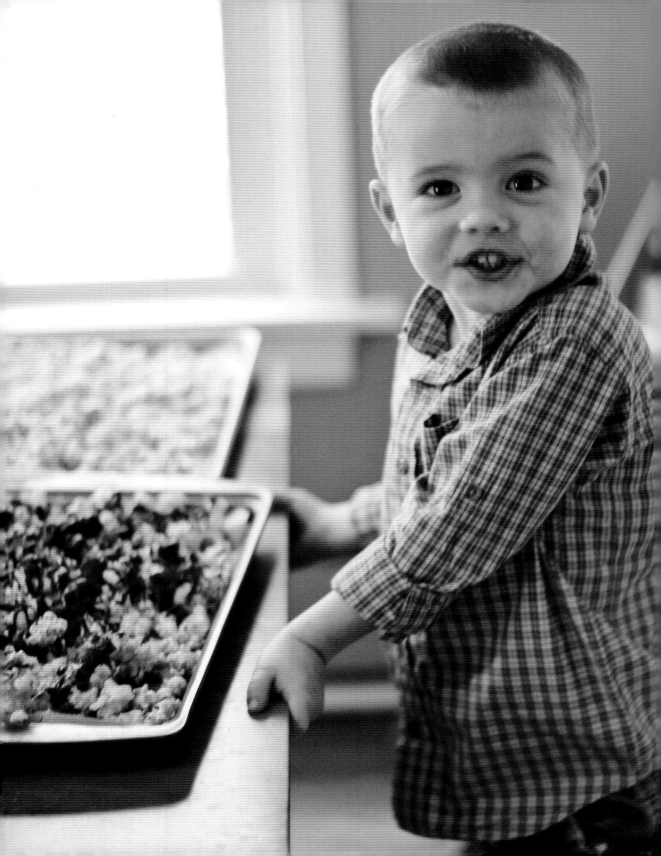

THE FOOD ALLERGY MAMA'S
Ways to Learn More and Give Back

There are many wonderful organizations dedicated to raising awareness about food allergies and providing funding for food allergy research. We've come a long way, but we still have more work to do.

A portion of the proceeds from *The Food Allergy Mama's Baking Book* will go to the Chicago chapter of the Food Allergy Initiative (FAI), an organization that was founded in 2007 by a group of parents dedicated to helping raise awareness of food allergies. FAI raises funds for food-allergy research. It is also committed to educating and training schools, day care centers, and camps about food allergies.

Another great way to directly impact food allergy research is to participate in a groundbreaking research initiative funded by the Bunning Food Allergy Institute at Children's Memorial Hospital in Chicago (see page 166 to learn how to participate). This wide-reaching study will look at the impact of environmental and genetic factors on children with food allergies.

There are still too many people out there who aren't aware of the dangers of food allergies. The more people know, the safer our children will be. It is my hope that, together, we can help to raise awareness about food allergies and someday find a cure.

The following is a list of great organizations that provided me with lots of helpful information when I needed it most.

Foundations and Professional Organizations

American Academy of Allergy, Asthma, and Immunology

555 East Wells Street
Milwaukee, WI 53202-3823
www.aaaai.org

American College of Allergy, Asthma, and Immunology

85 West Algonquin Road
Suite 550
Arlington Heights, IL 60005
800-842-7777
www.allergy.mcg.edu

American Medical Association

515 North State Street
Chicago, IL 60610
www.ama-assn.org

Asthma and Allergy Foundation of America

1233 20th Street, NW
Ste 402
Washington, DC 20036
www.aafa.org

Children's Memorial Food Allergy Study

To participate in this groundbreaking research initiative, contact Deanna Caruso by phone at 312-573-7755 or by e-mail at dcaruso@childrensmemorial.org.

The Elliot and Roslyn Jaffe Food Allergy Institute Mount Sinai School of Medicine

Box 1198
One Gustave L. Levy Place
New York, NY 10029
http://www.mssm.edu/jaffe_food_allergy

Food Allergy and Anaphylaxis Network

11781 Lee Jackson Highway
Suite 160
Fairfax, VA 22033-3309
www.foodallergy.org

Food Allergy Initiative Chicago

205 West Wacker Drive
Suite 1400
Chicago, IL 60606
http://www.faiusa.org/?page=chicago
FAIChicago@faiusa.org

Food Allergy Initiative National

1414 Avenue of the Americas
Suite 1804
New York, NY 10019
www.faiusa.org

The Illinois Food Allergy Association

181 Waukegan Road
Suite 306
Northfield, IL 60093
www.illinoisfaea.org

Medic Alert Jewelry and Pharmaceuticals MedicAlert Foundation

2323 Colorado Avenue
Turlock, CA 95382
www.medicalert.org

Mothers of Children Having Allergies (MOCHA)

www.mochallergies.org
info@mochallergies.org

Acknowledgments

I am grateful to so many people who helped make this book possible: first and foremost, my son John, who inspires me every day to not only bake great allergen-free treats but also to teach others about food allergies. Chloe, Matthew, and David, and especially my loving husband, Mike, provided the unwavering support and love I needed to get through the long days and nights of baking, testing, and writing. Without your patience and willingness to taste every single allergen-free treat, this book could not have been completed. I especially thank my amazing sister, Christina Stephens. You are my best friend and biggest cheerleader.

A huge thank you to Doug Seibold, president of Agate Publishing, for believing in my book and providing unlimited support and guidance. Perrin Davis and Eileen Johnson at Agate are also incredibly talented and a true joy to work with.

Thanks also go to Robert Knapp, the visionary who photographed all the beautiful shots in this book—your eye for style and substance is unmatched.

Thank you, Mark Czerniec, for creating and maintaining www.foodallergymama.com. Your tech expertise is far reaching, and I rely heavily on your talent.

Thank you, Linda Frothingham, for designing the Food Allergy Mama logo and Website; you captured my visions perfectly.

An enormous thanks to Kim and Scott Holstein; you've mentored and motivated me from day one, giving me the courage to think this was possible in the first place.

Thanks also to my amazing neighbors on Wilmette Avenue: the Browns, Carletons, Phelans, and Yamaguchis. Your constant willingness to taste-test my allergen-free creations is truly appreciated. You always opened your doors and hearts to my children when they dropped off baked goods on your doorstep, and I can't imagine this book being what it is without your great sense of taste.

To my family and friends, near and far, thank you for your limitless support, guidance, and advice.

Finally, a very big thank you goes to Dave and Denise Bunning for paving the way to food allergy awareness and research, and whose tireless work on behalf of food-allergic families is inspiring. I hope that, someday, food allergy mamas everywhere will get to see the day when food allergies are a thing of the past.

Index

About the Author

Kelly Rudnicki is the creator of the blog foodallergymama.com. The mother of four children, Rudnicki lives in suburban Chicago and spends much of her time promoting food allergy awareness. She has also worked as a television news producer and in corporate public relations. This is her first book.

GRAYSLAKE AREA PUBLIC LIBRARY
100 Library Lane
Grayslake, IL 60030